brazilbook
a division of brazildisc entertainment
chicago, il usa

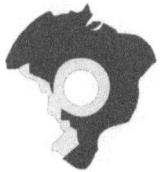

brazildisc

Donna's Song

Raymond O. West

Library of Congress information:

West, Raymond O., 1946-
Donna's Song – 1st ed. in the United States of America
p. cm.
ISBN-13: 978-1518871979
ISBN-10: 1518871976
Printed in the United States of America
10 9 8 7 6 5 4 3 2 1

To the memory of Donna,
her special gift,
and her life.

Prologue

I was blessed with the most glorious 35 years anyone could ever dream of. I was Donna's husband, lover, companion, and best friend. We met as teenagers, married young, suffered separation and the tempering of fire that war brings, and birthing a child while a husband is absent. But, we grew together. We often chided each other that we'd raised one another, and that we'd each done a good job.

I will concede that she raised me. I question that I raised her. She was born a gracious, loving person who in turn taught me how to love. She began by teaching me to love myself. I grew into loving others. Loving her was the easiest thing in life. We raised two children, both boys, to become extraordinary husbands, and one the father of three.

I am alone now. My beloved Donna has died. My anchor is no longer, and I find myself adrift, little but my words to distract me or comfort me. Donna was the one who patiently read every page of every manuscript I ever wrote, long before I submitted to any editor. At least until this one. Actually, there was one just before this one, a novella that I wrote to exorcise my pain. I had meant to read it to her, but by the time it was done, she was beyond hearing it or comprehending it. She had elicited a promise from me, in the weeks before she died, that I would write a book about her and her dying. The novella was meant to fulfill that promise to her, but turned out to be more of a release for me. So, now I write this, *Donna's Song,* in her honor and memory, and to fulfill the promise.

This is told in the first person. We shared deeply and honestly, throughout her (our) ordeal, as with our whole lives, and I feel safe that this is what she would have written, had she been able. She kept me focused, honest, and on track. This was written without her physical participation, but entirely with her inspiration. It is my greatest hope that it tells of her and her dying in such a way as to accomplish what she wanted. She asked that I never forget her, and I ask that you don't either.

Chapter One

"My nana has no hair," granddaughter Lucy announced to her friend and neighbor, Benjamin. Both five-year olds stood in front of me as I sat on the couch in my son's home, there for a visit with his family.

Both children continued to regard me with some curiosity, tilting their heads first to one side, and then the other. After some time, Lucy finally expanded on her observations. "My nana can't write," she added, just as matter-of-factly.

They stood there, quiet and polite, but curious, for some minutes more, before going about their more important business of playing.

It's true. I can't write. Or at least I can't write anything anyone could possibly read. What was once beautiful handwriting has become chicken scratches, and it's not something I'm happy about. I have lung cancer, and while I've been living with it or it with me, for a year now, I'm never prepared for what the next day or stage of the disease will visit on me. The hair loss is temporary, and has been coming back since chemotherapy ended. It's not the pretty hair I used to have. It's gray and fragile, but it's hair. My fatigue has improved as well with the abatement of radiation therapy. But the handwriting, that's a new twist.

In spite of best efforts, my cancer has spread. Now, tiny clusters of cancer cells reside in various parts of my left brain, and my right hand won't do what I want it to anymore. Neither will my right leg, or even my right eye. So, like Lucy says, nana can't write anymore.

Non small-cell lung cancer. Adenocarcinoma. Trouble is, it doesn't just stay in the lung. It moves around and spreads and shares its effects with most parts of the body. It's a scary, frustrating, dreaded highway I find myself on now, and there are no detours, no exits, and ever fewer rest stops. But it's not all gloom and doom either. I've got a family who loves me, and friends who care. I also have some family who hasn't been of any help at all. In fact, they've been of great harm, and it's been hard to learn how to separate from them. Most friends have been more than super. Only a very few have retreated from me, not knowing how to deal with it all. Well, guess what? I haven't known how to deal with it either, each step along the way. It's been new for me too.

So, what I want to do now is share something about what I've learned so it won't be quite so new to you. I want you not to be quite as afraid as I've been. You need a few key tools to do this job of living with cancer. Not a lot, but very important ones: a loving care-taker, a supportive family, lots of positive energy, understanding from both yourself and others, and a realization that life is a journey of unknown length and course. You don't need self-delusion, false hope and promises, or pity from anyone. Make it clear what you expect, and people will be amazingly cooperative.

So, let's look at the journey I've made so far. I'll pick a starting point of last great discovery and adventure, of freedom from pain and fear. It will help you know the sudden turn life takes when Adenocarcinoma becomes a part of your life.

I always thought of myself as a small town girl. Not well traveled, though I'd been married and living in a country outside my birthplace for the past 34 years. I'd grown up in a small out-port town on the coast of Newfoundland, and hadn't been any further away than the province's capital of St. John's until marrying. So, this trip was new to me, exciting and frightening. But, it was important to me, and my husband, and now it had begun.

As I looked out the window of the plane, watching the green coast change to blue ocean, I could feel my heart pounding. I felt lightheaded, not so much from the increased heart rate, but from the excitement that had built from the first time we'd talked of this trip.

It was mid-May, late afternoon, and the jumbo jet cut through the bright sky, racing away from the sun, carrying us to London, and the first leg of our trip to Bulgaria.

"I wonder if Jeremy is as excited as we are," I asked my husband, turning to face him.

He squeezed my hand, smiled. "You know he is."

And I knew he was. He'd been planning for our arrival since that day in January when we told him we were coming. We wanted to go to see where he lived and how. Each time we'd gotten a letter or phone call or even email, I painted a picture in my mind's eye of how things looked there, to him, where he was and what surrounded him. I'd wondered about his apartment, where it fit in the town where he lived, and how much like home it was. Jeremy had changed our itinerary around several times, and announcing the new plans with enthusiasm. He was as anxious to share his home as we were to see it. And all of us were anxious about his new love, Kristina. He was anxious to show her off, and we were anxious to meet her. I could well imagine how she felt about it all. I clearly remember when I first traveled to the states and met Ray's family. Poor Kristina, I thought to myself.

Even the cramped coach seats of the 747, and the long night that stretched out ahead of us, couldn't squelch the joy that rose from my chest, lit my face.

"I can't wait to see him." I settled back in my seat, wanting to sleep away the hours between now and then. "I wonder what Kristina is like."

"She's sounded beautiful on the phone," Ray answered. "And Jeremy sounds happy."

I didn't open my eyes, but nodded my agreement. "I hope she likes us."

The soft warmth of Ray's hand and the throbbing pulse of the engines that passed through the plane joined to comfort me into a light sleep.

Heathrow. The name sounded distant, larger than life, like a place I'd never visit. Yet, I watched the terminal come into view as the plane taxied into the gate. Heathrow: the stepping-off point for Eastern Europe.

Separate lines formed from the mass of passengers that descended on Customs and Immigration. My commonwealth passport put me in one line, my husband Ray, an American citizen, had his own line. It was all quick, simple, and we were together again, searching the crowd for a card bearing our name, held by our driver who would take us to Chadwick Airport, on the other side of London, and our connecting flight to Sofia. We'd been stacked up in air traffic for forty-five minutes, and the connection would be very close. But we made it, barely, rushing to the gate before the bus left, carrying all the passengers, and us across acres of concrete to our plane. We were halfway there.

The Alps stretched out below us, and the excitement inside me was building even further. I pictured how it would be, seeing my youngest son after so long a time. I rehearsed what I would say, and how I would say it. I imagined meeting Kristina, and wrote the words in my mind that I would use to greet her, to welcome her. Or, the words I would use to accept her welcome to her country. It was exhilarating to imagine it all.

Compared to Washington DC, and especially London, the tarmac seemed deserted. Only two planes were visible from my vantage point, straining to see this strange new land through the small portal of the plane. And, these were parked away from the terminal. No others were at what appeared to be the only gate, and none queued up behind us. But, the passengers that deplaned from our single flight rushed the Immigration counter of the Sofia Airport like a mob, and we ended up in the back, and a wait that seemed forever.

Minutes, that seemed like hours, later, we were through, pushing up the slight incline of steps, searching the sea of faces for Jeremy's. I felt panicked. I was so anxious to see him. And then, there he was, smiling over the railing above, waving down at me. Tears streamed down my cheeks, and I ran. Ran to see my son, hold my baby, mother and comfort him. Ran to make up for the long, endless stream of time that had kept us apart.

He was there, well and waiting, and now pushing through the crowd toward me to shorten the distance. Jeremy was taller than Ray, with thinning blonde hair, piercing blue eyes, and handsome in the same way that his father was handsome: rugged and independent, strong and silent, reassuring and strong.

All the things I'd thought about saying on the plane, rehearsed in my mind, when I had him back again were gone. I couldn't say anything. I could only wrap my arms around him, and sob with joy.

"Mom, Dad, I want you to meet Kristina," Jeremy said. He was bursting with pride, glowing as he looked to her.

Ray had been right. She was beautiful. And, my son was as happy as I'd ever seen him.

We spent that next week touring Bulgaria with Jeremy and Kristina. This had been Jeremy's Peace Corps assignment for the past two years, and it had been that long since I'd done no more than talk to him on the phone, or read his emails. It was unreal to see this son of mine guide us so skillfully and confidently around his new world. He was fluent in the language, adept at their ways and comfortable with their culture: his new culture. He took enormous pride in this country, and of his Kristina. I watched him with her and her with him, and saw Ray and myself, as we were all those years before, when we dated in my native Newfoundland.

Sofia was a crowded city, with stone paved streets, narrow, lined with shops and walkup apartments. I had never seen such old buildings, streets, and ancient excavations below the streets that developers had worked into the design of their modern plans.

We spent two wonderful days in Sofia, visiting the czar's palace, cafes, and museums. We stayed in a third floor apartment converted into a small hotel, with four separate sleeping rooms and a single bath. It was comfortable, but I worried when Jeremy and Kristina would leave us at night, headed back to her apartment. The innkeeper spoke no English, and there was no way we could have addressed any problem.

Next we went to Plovdiv, taking a bus from Sofia south and east to the country's cultural center, with a modern skyline dotted with minarets, streets wide and pedestrian. The traffic jams of Sofia, and the world's other cities, were held away to the edges of the city, and we walked on stone roads built by Romans two thousand years earlier. We sat in cafes in the city's heart, and looked up at the hill in the city's core at Old Plovdiv. We walked there, and toured the houses and buildings of hundreds of years ago, feeling the special magic of lives long gone. Gardens lined walls that blocked out the cobble-stoned streets and served as moats to protect the grand, but aging, houses. Jeremy bartered with an old woman, buying me a hand woven table doily that would dwarf our dining room table. Ray bought a Russian doll, beautifully painted with eight little identical sisters tucked neatly inside, progressively smaller.

We toured the monuments and cathedrals, palaces and squares, parks and theatres, and every where there were blooms and children playing and old men strolling, capped by their berets and holding their canes. Street vendors sold books, old tomes and new, art books, music books, travel and language books. Musicians played for coins, and serious seniors huddled over chessboards in the city's most central park.

In those two days, we took a bus trip to see a monastery, perched on a hillside by a road that ran along the path of a large river. Murals decorated the ceilings and walls, vines covered the walls and exotic trees and shrubs grew lush in the gardens.

Ray and I talked about how wonderful it would be to live in a city like Plovdiv, with cafes for morning tea and rolls, lunches under canvas awnings, watching brightly garbed people bustle by, doing the tasks that gave them meaning.

Ray became sick in Plovdiv. Ray never got sick, not so much as a cold, yet on the third day of this wondrous adventure, he lost his voice, his throat swelled nearly shut, his chest hurt with sharp darting pains. I worried so for him. Pharmacies were everywhere, and sold anything you knew to ask for. We bought codeine and syrups and pills to reduce his temperature and raspy cough. I really think there were a couple of days and side trips that he missed completely. Not because he didn't go with us, but because he was so sick and miserable that he didn't know or care where he was. The misery stayed with him for several days, costing him some joy.

Then we moved on to our final destination, spending three days in Etropole, the small city in the Balkan Mountains where Jeremy lived and worked. We stayed with him and Kristina in his small apartment, met his friends, saw the market where he bought food, the restaurant where he'd entertain Kristina when she'd visit from Sofia, and walked the streets and hiked the hillsides. We met his co-workers, and with Jeremy and Kristina translating, found out what they thought of our son, and America, and we thanked them for the way they all watched over him.

Doncho, Jeremy's best friend in the forestry offices, invited us to his home where his wife and two daughters entertained us with a traditional Bulgarian feast; Naghosti, it's called. Their stucco house was across town, and we walked carrying the flowers and candy that were traditional hostess gifts. The streets were tree lined, with no sidewalks, and carried us through the central market, past small office and official buildings, an outdoor bar nestled under trees, and houses with small private gardens instead of lawns. The locals we passed stared politely at the exceptional strangers in their town.

We ate slowly, enjoying each course of the meal, and drank wine and Rakeya, the homemade liquor that was thick and strong. It was nearly midnight when we got back to Jeremy's apartment.

I bonded with Kristina that week. Bonded in a way only someone who'd married a love from far away could bond with a woman who was so apparently in love with some one new and young from even further away.

It was a wonderful week that ended too soon.

Jeremy came with us to England. He'd been there before, and was anxious to see things he'd missed, and we welcomed his experience. Watching him and Kristina saying goodbye as he left her behind in Sofia, even for a week, reminded me of the past sadness I'd felt when Ray had had to say goodbye to me over the years. My heart ached for her.

From London, the three of us flew to Dublin. My favorite television show for some time had been Balleykissangel, a PBS broadcast based in a quaint Irish village. Its cast of characters had become a family to me, and with the ending of each episode, I would tearfully wish to be in Balleykissangel, never mind that it was fictional. Somehow Ray had discovered that it was filmed in a real town, Avoca, some 100 kilometers southwest of Dublin. He arranged a great surprise for me, and by train and bus he took us there.

I walked the streets I so dreamed of being a part of, visited Fitzgerald's Pub, the church, the little food market, and stood on the stone arched bridge above the stream at the entrance of town. I strained to see my favorite characters that I expected to see walk along beside the stone walls or step out through a low wood door. It was during a break in filming there, so no one was about but us tourists. Still, it was heaven. Too soon we had to return to London and prepare for our return home.

Jeremy left the morning we did, but two hours earlier. I held him tight, knowing that in just five months I would have him home again. It was hard, watching him walk away down the street in London toward the train station. Ray was finally himself again, free from his sudden and painful illness, and I felt happy.

Fulfilling my fantasy, seeing my beautiful son and meeting his equally beautiful love, sharing this magical two weeks with my love: it was all so wonderful I didn't want it to end. I couldn't know then that it would make for the last great memory of my life.

Chapter Two

We were early into that summer of 2001 when we returned home. Ray went to the doctor, concerned with the lingering symptoms of whatever it was that had infected him in Bulgaria. His chest x-ray was clear, but the doctor prescribed some powerful antibiotics to thoroughly clear his system.

For my part, I had begun to develop a tickle deep at the top of my chest. I coughed to relieve it, loosen it, but it stayed. This dry, throat-clearing cough was becoming part of my day. I tried to suppress the concern I had. A childhood friend who'd ended up living close by, had died last year of breast cancer, and what I'd noticed most in the last year of her life was a soft, constant cough. A shiver of fear ran through me, but I pushed it aside. Not completely, though. It stayed there close to the surface like a dark cloak that threatened to envelop me, but whenever I felt the panic, I forced it away in a corner and tried to ignore it.

At Ray's insistence, I called our doctor. She was on vacation, but her partner saw me, told me it was allergies, and to be patient, use some lozenges and honey syrup with tea.

That summer, I shared the photos of our trip with anyone I could pin down. I talked endlessly about Jeremy, Kristina, Bulgaria and Avoca: Balleykissangel. Everyone especially liked the photo Ray had taken of me sitting in Fitzgerald's Pub, at my favorite characters' regular table, with a pint of Guinness.

That summer, I planned for Jeremy's homecoming in early October. I started marking the calendar each day, tracking the time until we'd meet him at the airport.

June yielded to July, and then August. The dry, irritating cough became a constant. I hadn't remembered pollen or allergies ever having this much of an effect on me. By the end of August, Ray prodded me to go back to the doctor. His pet name for me is *baby girl*.

"Baby girl," he said. "I worry about you. That can't be just allergies. There's something else wrong. Please, see our regular doctor. Promise?"

I made an appointment for the first week of September, insisting on my regular doctor, Suzanne Ross. She examined me carefully, and ordered chest x-rays. It would be a week or so, she promised, and they'd call with any results.

The horror of September 11 filled our lives for just one week. All I could think about in those few days was Jeremy, overseas and vulnerable. I wanted him home, protected. It made me forget about pending radiology readings, the cough, and the subtle changes taking place in the look of my eyes reflected in the mirror.

The doctor's office finally called, and I scheduled an appointment for September 18. Ray met me at home. He wanted to go with me, and came by from work to pick me up. It was the middle of the month, and what was most on my mind was October first, getting Jeremy home, and the fear we all lived under, waiting for the next terrorist attack and hoping it would never come. Ray stayed in the waiting room when the nurse called my name.

"Is your husband with you?" Dr. Ross asked as she came into the examination room. The wait had been short this visit. I'd barely settled in the small plastic chair, hadn't had the time to get uncomfortable yet.

"Yes, he's in the waiting room," I replied. "Why?"

"I'd like to discuss this with the two of you. Let me have the nurse get him," she responded. She avoided looking directly at me, flipping back and forth through the pages of my chart.

A terror gripped me. A cold, numbing terror shocked my heart, then spread out through my arms and legs, pushing up to my head, making my neck spasm and my head jerk. Horrible fears filled my thoughts; dread consumed me. In all my fifty-five years no doctor had ever delayed a test result for someone else to be there. I'd never had to wait until Ray was with me to have a doctor share news of anything. I imagined the worst, and knew it was going to be. The fear I had about my friend's death had never really gone away, but now it wouldn't stay pushed into the dark recesses of my consciousness. Now it was right in front of me, screaming at me, scaring me.

By the time the door opened, and Ray hesitantly came into the room, I was in tears. He stood there, at first confused then frightened, looking from me to Dr. Ross, and back to me.

Dr. Ross stood quietly, hesitant, uncomfortable. "This is what I hate most about medicine," she said, so quietly it went almost unheard.

I looked at Ray, blurry from my tears, wanting him to make things right again.

"I'm afraid it's not good," the doctor was saying. Ray and I looked numbly at each other. "If it is malignant, and I think it is, it's not a good cancer to have."

I can't remember the rest of that day. Ray had made an appointment for me that Tuesday in the hospital's radiology department, where they would do a biopsy, sticking a long needle deep in my lung. Ray was trying to be upbeat, reminding me that the results weren't in yet, and that even if it were the worst, enormous strides had been made in treatments, that I would be okay. The doctor's caution that it wasn't a good cancer to have crashed around in my mind, and suddenly I couldn't see myself growing old. I couldn't see myself sharing in Ray's life, or watching my grandchildren grow up, or Jeremy marry Kristina, if that's what they decided to do. Somehow, I knew I wouldn't survive, but I kept that from Ray.

The world's war with terrorists receded to the most remote part of my mind, maybe leaving it all together. I had my own terrorist to deal with now.

I didn't want to let go of Ray's hand. I was lying on the gurney, in the hallway, with tranquilizers being fed into me with the intravenous tubing that was supposed to sedate me, but I felt panic. The bright lights in the ceiling made me feel exposed and alone, and without his company I didn't think I could survive. Masked, gray-gowned figures were at the foot and head of the gurney, and they were urging me to let go of Ray's hand. It slipped away, my fingers losing touch, and they pushed me through doors and down a hall, into a room with more people masked and robed. A rubber mask went over my face, and I slipped away into the fluid dark place that I hadn't been to since Jeremy was born.

I dreamed in this dark, familiar again place, of glowing golden lights and soft breezes bathing me in their wash. I dreamed of being far away, missing Ray, pulled to a star in a far corner of the universe. Time stopped in this new place, new life, and while I was alone there, I felt submerged in a sea of others. The gentle tide pool held me afloat and gently raised me up and down. The pleasantness calmed me, made me want to stay, as I became aware of lights and pressure in my chest.

A soothing voice pushed through my ear and into my consciousness.

"Baby girl, it's okay. It's over."

I let my eyes drift slowly open, not wanting the world to engulf this peace. But the light and cold and dull ache in my lung woke me up. Ray was standing by the gurney, back in the hall, his face close to mine, and his hand holding mine. I woke to his eyes looking close at me; their usual blue calm troubled.

"Oh, sweetie. I didn't think I was coming back," I said.

"Back from where?" Ray asked.

Already the strange place I'd been to began to dissolve, to disappear, and to fly away from my memory. "I'm not sure now."

The doctor who'd taken the biopsy came to us, and told us that the results would be ready Friday, and that our doctor would contact us for an appointment. He went on with instructions in case my lung collapsed, but I couldn't hear what he was saying. His words were noises. Ray would listen and know what to do.

We made a deal that I would stay home from work Friday, and Dr. Ross would call Ray at his work with the results. He'd come home then, and tell me. I couldn't bear the thought of hearing it in the clinical offices, and I wanted to hear it from Ray.

I watched through the window all morning, nervously hoping Ray would pull in the driveway, and hoped that he wouldn't. I wanted the time to go fast so the wait would be over, but I wanted time to stop so that I would never have to hear. It was just before noon when Ray's Jeep turned in off the street.

I stood frozen at first in the living room, afraid to go to the door, hoping to see something in Ray's eyes or walk or something that would give me a hint. Instead, he walked toward the house with a steady walk and eyes that showed no agony. So, I went to the door, opened it and leaned out, looking at him for hope, and feeling only dread.

"I love you, baby girl," he said. He wrapped his arms around me and held me tight. "Whatever comes now, I'm with you. All the way. You won't be alone, I promise."

I couldn't help it. My chest began to heave and tears filled my eyes, spilling out on Ray's shoulder. I started to shake all over, and felt the life force drain from me.

We spent that afternoon together, at first quiet, just holding each other. As hard as he tried not to, Ray cried with me. It's true what they say. Your whole life rolls past in front of you like a movie when you face death. Sitting there on the sofa, holding tight to Ray and being held, everything I'd ever done or felt or thought in my life played out in front of me.

"What happens now?" I finally managed. "What do we do?"

"Dr. Ross gave us several options for referrals," Ray said. "Her husband was one of them, Basil Yanis, and he can see you Monday.

"I've checked around, and he's got a good reputation as an Oncologist. He's a department head at the hospital, and we know some people who've been his patients." Ray hesitated. "We're on new ground here, baby girl, and I think time is important. You want me to make the appointment?"

"Will you go with me?"

Ray tightened the hold he already had me in. His lips brushed my ear, cheek, then lightly crossed my lips. He pulled his head back slightly, so we could focus on each other. His eyes looked intensely into mine.

"You won't be alone for a single thing that happens from now on," he said softly. "Do you understand?"

Fear gripped me again, and the shaking in my neck started again. I couldn't help it or stop it. I managed a nod, then dropped my head back on Ray's shoulders, sobbing. He held me, firmly and gently, and rocked me slightly. I knew he understood because he didn't try to say anything, or hurry me along or do anything but hold me close for as long as I wanted.

Ray called in for me at work, telling my boss Ryan that he had to take me to a specialist that afternoon. He went on to work, promising to be home for lunch and the appointment. I stayed in bed, trying to hide under the blanket and comforter. As a little girl, I'd slept under piles of quilts and comforters, crushing me with their warmth and pushing away the cold winter nights of Newfoundland. It always made me feel warm and secure, and I wanted that feeling back again.

I dreamed without sleeping. It was growing dark and my toes were numb. We skated around the pond, laughing and chasing each other. My brother Jim played hockey with the other boys, and we girls watched them closely, pretending not to, and giggling with each other. The world seemed safe and warm, in spite of the piercing cold.

"Can't we play more?" I cried. My father lifted me up, tucked me under his arm, and carried me home, my feet and hands too frozen to take off my skates.

I turned my head, and looked at the alarm clock. It was nearly eleven and Ray would be home soon. I pushed the blankets off me and sat up, trying to gain the strength and balance to get out of bed, get showered and dressed. I was suspended between my dream memories and now.

I stared closely at the eyes looking back from the mirror. What happened, I wondered? I hadn't paid attention to the changes in this reflection, until now. How could things go this wrong? I pushed the comb of the hairdryer though my hair, and watched myself intently. It was like looking at a stranger's face, somehow detached. I felt detached, like I was living some kind of dream. The acrid taste of fear crept into my throat and the back of my mouth. My hand started shaking. The eyes in the mirror filled with tears and streamed down this stranger's face.

The waiting room was full of people who had no hair. There were children, young people, and a pregnant young woman holding hands with her boyish husband. A scarf covered her head, and the smooth skin of her face went up behind her ears and under the scarf where her hair should have been.

"Madonna West?" the nurse called out from the doorway leading into the hallway of the inner workings of the clinic.

I tightened my grip on Ray's hand, and looked at him, pleading mutely to make this stop.

"I'm with you, baby girl," he said. He stood, helped me up, and guided me toward the nurse.

"We need to get some blood work first," the nurse said. "You can sit here." She pointed Ray to a chair by the door to the lab. I wouldn't be out of his sight, so I let go of his hand, and let the nurse lead me to my chair. I didn't even feel the needle, and it seemed like no time at all had passed and the nurse was leading us to the examination room.

"Mrs. West," the nurse asked. She shut the door behind her and motioned for Ray and me to sit down. "Do you prefer to be called Madonna, or Donna?"

"Donna."

"Donna, I'm Judy, Dr. Yanis's nurse. You're in good hands now."

She took my blood pressure; made notes in the chart she'd sat on the table, and turned to face us.

"Don't feel like you're alone in this," she said gently. She was short, a little older than me, wore glasses, and had a friendly, comforting way about her. "We'll help you in any way we can. We've got a lot of experience."

"What comes next?" Ray asked.

"The doctor will go over your treatments with you. He'll be here in just a few minutes." She pulled the door open, stepping out into the hallway. "If you need anything, just open the door and call out."

We were alone in the small room, and I looked at Ray, terror filling my heart. He reached across to my knee, and I put my hand on his. "I don't want to do this."

"I know, baby girl," he answered. He said this softly, really knowing my fears. "But this is important. This is what will keep you with me." He turned his hand over and squeezed it around mine. His mouth smiled, but his eyes didn't. They seemed so alone and frightened, mirrors of my own.

The door opened and I lost my breath.

Basil Yanis was a little younger than either Ray or me. His white smock was buttoned tightly around his front, and glasses perched on the end of his nose. He sat down on the stool across from us, opened my chart, and scanned the pages, flipping from one sheet to the next, then back again. After what seemed an endless time, he looked up.

"We'll start you this week with chemotherapy," he said simply. "It will be mixed with radiation treatment for the next couple of months."

He continued to talk. His lips moved and his eyes looked from me to Ray as he spoke, but I couldn't hear the words. It was a droning noise that gradually slipped away to mute. I stared at him, but really through him and past him. Time had stopped again.

"We're only in our fifties," I heard Ray say, snapping me out of the trance I had put myself in. "We want to know we have a long time left together."

Dr. Yanis smiled thinly, and shook his head no.

"A decade at least?" Ray asked.

Again, a thin smile and a nod that no, such time wasn't there.

"How long?" Ray finally asked, the frustration and fear apparent in his voice.

"It's all theory," the doctor answered. "You may have several years left. We'll do everything we can with what is available."

I felt myself drift away again, but heard some talk from the doctor about what kind of cancer it was, what kind of chemicals he'd use in treatment, what kind of problems awaited me, what kind of time I might have left. But none of it made real sense to me. I couldn't allow myself to focus on what he was saying.

I came back to the room with the squeeze Ray was giving my hand. "Are you alright?"

I looked numbly at him, trying to focus my eyes. "What?"

Ray turned in his chair to face me, taking my hand with both of his. "Are you alright?"

I felt the crushing fear and tears rise up from deep in my chest. I fought for control, but couldn't and instead began sobbing with jagged breaths. Ray leaned into me, put his arms around me, and rocked me like he had the day he'd come home to tell me the results of the test. My life was over, and I knew it. It must feel like this to drown, I thought, as I fought for breath.

Neither of us said anything as Ray drove us away from the hospital toward home. We hadn't said anything to anyone in the days since the diagnosis. Without discussion, Ray had picked up the cell phone and had called our oldest son.

"Listen, son," Ray began. "There's no easy way to tell you this. I need you to sit down and listen carefully." He looked over to me but I couldn't bear to meet his gaze. "We've just come from the doctor."

Ray faltered, his eyes filling with tears that he fought back. He swallowed hard and started again. "Mom has cancer, Raymond." His breath came jagged then, and he stopped talking. I looked over at him, and his face was consumed with a distant, hollow expression. Tears ran down his cheek. He tried again, but started crying before he could speak.

"I'm sorry, Raymond," he finally managed. "This is so hard."

"No, son, it's certain," he said after a long silence. "We've known for a week. We were just at the oncologist and got the treatment schedule that starts Wednesday."

He was quiet for a long time then, just holding the phone, listening.

"I'm sorry, Raymond, I'll have to call you back later," was all Ray could manage, then he set the phone down and grasped the wheel with both hands. His lips trembled as he drove down the street.

I imagined how our son had taken the news, wondered at what he'd said, wanted to know how he'd left it, but could only look through the window at the nothingness passing us by.

*****

We spent the morning in a classroom, part of the office area of the oncology clinic, Ray beside me with his hand on my knee, pressing reassuringly. A nurse was introducing the small class of new cancer patients to the chemotherapy regimen: various schedules of treatment, mixes of toxins that would be pumped into us and through us. I looked around the small room at the three other patients at the table. An older lady sat with her daughter holding her hand. Two other women sat by themselves, one my age, and the third woman much younger than me. Her cancer was in her breast, the two others in their lymph systems. I was the only lung cancer patient. The nurse talked positively to them about what success they could expect. She offered no such assurances to me. Mine was the cancer not talked about in the group.

Each of us was led separately from the classroom, down the hall to the other wing of the floor, to the treatment area. Ray went with me for my tour, and I leaned heavily on his arm. The room was lined with recliners, I.V. poles stationed by each. The few patients there for treatment were either sleeping or reading while clear bags of chemicals drained into their bodies through needles in their arms. One woman wore a scarf to cover her nearly bald head, and a man with a ball cap had smooth, pale skin around the bottom of the cap. They all looked fragile.

I looked at Ray, the panic in my eyes reflecting what I felt in my chest. I tried to speak, but couldn't, the sound choking off in my throat. He didn't look at me, but held tight to my arm as he scanned the room with me.

"We don't like care-takers to be in the treatment room during chemotherapy," the nurse was saying. "But, we want you both to see what it's like." Her voice and manner were soft. "Donna," she continued, turning her attention to just me, "I'll be your treatment nurse. Which chair would you like?"

The soft green vinyl of the chairs was identical, with half of them facing the windows at the back of the room, and the other half backed up under the windows. All of them seemed frightening.

"How long will I be here?" I finally managed.

"Each treatment will be about three hours," she answered.

I couldn't imagine sitting here that long, in any of the chairs. I watched as another nurse replaced an empty bag on one pole with another one bulging with clear fluid. Dr. Yanis had said that six different chemicals would be used for each of my treatments. Six different bags of

toxins changed and added to what would be pumped into my body twice a week for the next three months. I couldn't imagine sleeping during each of these visits, and the view through the window was the gray wall of the hospital across the street.

"Could I sit under a window?" I asked, imagining the light it would give me while I read those three long hours.

"Of course," she answered, smiling. "How about this one?"

I nodded my agreement, unable to speak. She led me to the one in the middle of the windowed wall, easing me out of Ray's firm grasp and guiding me into the chair.

"You can sit here for this treatment," she said, pointing Ray toward a small swivel stool by the foot of the chair. "It will be the only chance you have to join her as we progress."

Ray pulled the stool nearer the chair with his foot, and sat down, reaching over to hold my free hand while the nurse prepared my other arm for the needle she would push into my vein. I know that sadness and fear filled my face as I looked at Ray, trying not to think about what they were doing to me, what it all meant. I wanted to be brave for him, meet the upbeat mood he had been trying to bring into all this mess, but I couldn't. I choked back the tears that were ready to fill my eyes again.

Chapter Three

Jeremy came home from Bulgaria the first of October. It was the first good thing that had happened to me, to us, in the past month. When I'd last seen him in May, I had been filled with the hope that everything would be right side up again when he got home. Now here we were, waiting for him in the airport in Cincinnati, and everything was turned upside down.

We looked down over the railing toward the escalator where passengers were entering the terminal from the various gates, his flight number on the screens showing that his plane had landed. Jeremy didn't know about my cancer. We couldn't tell him from that far away. My excitement of seeing him lost to the over riding worry about my dying, and for Ray the dread of having to tell him.

When he did appear in the line of passengers, my heart leaped anyway, and he looked up to scan the sea of faces much as I had done months earlier in Sofia, looking for him. His face beamed when he saw us, and he waved and smiled.

It was joyous to have him here again, but the ride home was subdued. We listened as he talked, updating us on everything new in his life, everything new with Kristina. He seemed not to notice my quiet withdrawal. Ray did what he could to keep Jeremy talking and upbeat.

"You tell him," I pleaded as Jeremy settled into his old room. "I can't. I can't."

Ray nodded, and turned toward the hall, headed for Jeremy and what I knew was a dreaded talk. It seemed like only moments when I felt breathing by my side and turned to see my son looking at me with the saddest eyes he'd ever worn. He didn't speak, but turned me toward him, wrapped me with his arms, and told me that he loved me so. He cried as hard as I did.

We were a family again. Jeremy would live with us, find some work until fall, when he would go to graduate school. He'd applied only to a single place, Yale. I loved him for his self-confidence. I loved him for being here with me.

"I can smell the chemicals in your skin, baby girl," Ray said when we got home from the latest treatment. "You've got to feel lousy all the way through."

I was surprised that I didn't, really. This one had taken more than three hours, as most of them had. Each one since the first had been with him waiting in the sitting area outside treatment, and I struggled with having to do these without him by my side, but physically I didn't feel much different than before the treatment.

"I'm okay, really," I answered him. "I don't want to think about what the radiation will feel like, though." In two more days we'd meet for the first time with the radiation oncologist and find out what was planned. "I wish I could just stop this."

"Stop the cancer, yes," Ray replied. "I wish we could stop the rest too, but you know we can't."

"I know," I answered. "I just want you to hold me now."

He pulled me tight to him. I was afraid with the changes happening inside me, the chemicals that had left their smell with me, he wouldn't want to be close. I was glad for the intimacy he showed as he nestled my face against him and stroked my back.

"We could make love, you know," I said, trying to smile as I gazed up at him. I needed to know he still wanted me that way, as a woman and lover. I wanted to know that I was still what I had been to him for the past 34 years. It had been a big part of our lives.

"In the middle of the afternoon?" he joked. But there was a twinkle in his eye as he turned us toward the bedroom. "Yeah, the middle of the afternoon. Sounds like fun!"

"I've got an MRI scheduled for tomorrow, you know," I said as we lay together, snuggling close. The aftermath of lovemaking had settled and my mind had turned back toward the thing that most ruled my thoughts.

"You want me to pick you up at work, or meet you at home?"

"Don't be silly," I said. I turned my face up to look at his, my cheek rubbing into his chest hair. "It's only a test, and it's near my office. I'll be fine."

"I told you that you wouldn't be alone for any of this," he said, looking down at my eyes with a serious expression. "I meant it."

"I know you did, sweetie, but this is simple. I can manage. Really."

Ray didn't push it, but I could see that he felt he should be there.

"You've missed enough work as it is," I went on, trying to assure him. "I can handle this just fine."

The next afternoon I sat alone in the waiting area of the medical testing clinic, waiting for the latest in the now constant round of testing and probing. My mind wandered far away from the bleak paneled walls of the room, back to my life that I loved without this awful, crushing weight on me. I could see the little town of Avaco as if I was there again, and feel the joy of seeing Jeremy's face in that sea of strangers in the Sofia airport. I was far away from the damning gloom of doctors and sickness.

I was startled out of my reverie by the telltale cracking of anklebones coming from the stairway leading down to the area I was in. I could always hear Ray coming that way, and I turned just in time to see him come around the landing and the final steps. He saw me immediately, and came and sat in the chair by me.

"Hi, baby girl," he said playfully, grabbing my hand and squeezing it.

"You don't need to be here," I admonished him, trying my best to look stern.

"Nothing alone from now on, remember?" he said, and smiled.

I tried to be serious, but couldn't. I was really glad to see him, to have him here.

"You can't go in, you know," I said.

"Don't have to," he answered. "Being here is fine. This way I can walk you to your car when you're done."

It made it harder, leaving him when they called my name. But I knew it would be easier coming out of the test. I leaned over and gave him a kiss as I got up.

*****

Rebecca Passen, the radiation oncologist, had been the doctor who'd ordered the MRI I had yesterday. And, as Ray and I sat with her in the hospital office, I was taken aback by how young she seemed. I liked her manner right away, and appreciated the straightforward way she was talking with us.

"It's a benchmark," she was saying. "I need to know exactly what size the tumor is, where it is precisely to mark the target settings for treatments. When we've finished this round of therapy, we'll order another MRI, then compare. She stood up as she pulled the X-rays from the folder, and snapped them in the clips of the lighted panel on the wall.

"Look at this," she offered. "This is the lung tumor we're treating primarily." She used her pen to point at the light area above my heart. "It's on the Aortic Arch, which is why we can't operate. And it's four centimeters long. In the next two months, we're hoping it will be smaller."

I felt like she'd already told me more than Dr. Yanis had, but I realized that I was beginning to pay more attention, beginning to want to know more.

"It seems so small," I said, gazing at the sphere of light area.

"It is, except as it relates to the lung," she replied. "It's really quite large for that environment."

As I peered at the X-ray, her comment about primary treatment hit me. "What do you mean by primary treatment?" I asked.

"Here," she said, pointing to a tiny spot on my spine, visible from the side view. "There's a small lesion here as well."

"Are we sure it's cancer too?" Ray asked, leaning over my shoulder, looking at the X-ray with me. "Will you do an autopsy on that?"

Dr. Passen pulled back from the panel. "No," she said. "We can't do that, but we can't take the risk it's being anything but another tumor. We're sure it is, and we'll treat it like one."

Suddenly panic set in again. I had nearly lost my reason considering a tumor in my lung, but this was not my lung. It was my spine. The image of the cancer spreading out like a fungus throughout my body slammed into my consciousness, and I staggered back, feeling faint.

Ray grabbed me, and eased me back into the chair.

"Already?" he asked weakly. "It's spread already?"

Dr. Passen kept her straightforward approach. "Metastasizing is the nature of this cancer particularly. Hopefully, this is all there is."

It hadn't occurred to either of us that there would be more, this early. We'd thought if all of this treatment and examination started soon enough, it wouldn't grow. We were neither one ready for this new information.

The treatments were in the hospital's radiology department, and we parked in the lot on the garage rooftop by the emergency room. It was a block or so long walk back to the treatment area. We checked in with the receptionist, and settled into chairs in the small hallway across from the desk.

"Wonder how this works?" Ray asked, nodding toward the elevator door at the end of the small hall.

"The treatment area's below by three floors," another patient across from us said. "It's shielded and remote. Gotta protect the hospital population," he finished with a snort.

The stainless steel doors looked foreboding, but I didn't have time to consider it all when the pager they'd given us at the desk went off. Ray took it back to the receptionist and came back for me.

"We're about to find out what's down there," he said, holding the elevator door for me while I stepped in.

The room at the other side of this ride looked as much like a living room as it could with its tiled floors and tiled ceilings. The furniture was comfortable and tasteful, and the plants gave it a calming feel. And, like every other step along the way in this nightmare, the staff was friendly and supportive. More than that; helpful, really. A young woman in pale green who introduced herself as my radiation therapist greeted us.

"I'll show you both the treatment area," she offered, turning to guide us down another hall. "You'll have to go back to the waiting area then, so we can get started," she said to Ray.

She measured me from several angles, referred to my chart, and made cross marks on my neck and chest. "These are my target points," she explained as she pressed the marker onto my skin. "And to make sure they don't wash off, I'm covering them with this special water proof tape."

She pressed the small sections of tape on my skin, over the marks, and had me lie still while she moved equipment along ceiling tracks over my head. The cool, subdued light was meant to be relaxing, I'm sure, but the panic set in again, and my body trembled.

Alone in the room, I did what I could to follow her instructions through the speaker outside the booth where she'd gone to operate the deadly radiation dosages. I was getting used to the probing and pressures and new sensations, but I didn't like them. It was over fast enough that I didn't have time to consider what was happening. It wasn't like the drawn out chemotherapy I'd begun in the weeks before. That seemed like a bonus.

"We'll have you back the day after tomorrow," she said, rejoining me in the room. She moved the equipment away from the table and helped me sit up. "Is this time good for you?"

Good for me, I thought. No time is good for me, I wanted to say. Instead, I asked, "Will it be as quick for the rest of the treatments?"

"Quicker," she answered. "With all the marks made, we just have to calibrate the equipment. It won't be more than a few minutes from now on."

Somehow, this seemed like a victory. I slid off the table, pulled the curtain back on the dressing area, and changed the hospital robe for my clothes.

"That didn't take long," Ray said as the therapist walked me back to the waiting area. He jumped up from his chair and slipped his arm around my shoulder. "Did it go okay?"

"Better than the chemo," I answered. "But, I'm ready to go home." It's amazing how such little things could tire me so. Maybe it was the cumulative effect of weeks of treatments; maybe it was the cancer. Maybe it was both. I didn't like this new tiredness that was taking me over.

The next weeks were a schedule of clinical visits for three-hour shifts of toxins, twice weekly radiation doses, and work when I could slip it in. Our home life became a retreat for rest and escape. I wanted normalcy there at any cost. It worked for awhile, until the end of the first month of chemotherapy, when I pulled a comb through my hair. I held it in my hand and lost my breath. The teeth were filled with hair. My hair. Long shiny strands of light brown. They fell off the comb and into the sink. I looked at the mirror to see what had been a thick mat of carefully shaped hair stick out in loose strands. What they'd promised was now happening, but I wasn't really prepared for it.

It had, in ways, seemed this horrible legacy had begun only moments before. That my normal life would resume soon, or that it was a short and horrible nightmare that would soon be interrupted. In other ways it had begun to seem like my whole life, that happiness and hope had preceded this stage many lifetimes ago. There were, assuredly, benchmarks along the way on this leg of my life's journey, but none had been so real, so inalterable, so scary as this comb full of hair. I had my vanities, though few, and my hair had always been one of them. Now, it was going and everything seemed more real, more permanent, and more deadly.

The week before, my coworker and good friend Nedra had heard me make an appointment at a wig shop that specialized in hair loss replacement for cancer patients. They'd had brochures in the oncology clinic, and with reminders each visit by the nurses and staff that I was lucky my hair was still holding, I'd begun to worry about the way I'd feel without it, how I'd look, and how I'd ever find a wig that matched exactly what it was to replace. We'd decided to take care of it before it was lost.

The next day, Ray and I had gone to pick out the wig that would be my hair until treatments stopped and mine would be allowed to grow back again. It was fun and silly, trying on wigs of different shapes and colors, teasing Ray and primping in front of the mirror. From what Ray called fantasy wigs, long and blond, to blends of gray and brown, and finally short waved auburn strands with highlights that most nearly matched my own, I made my selection, and we went to the counter to pay for it.

"That's already taken care of," the lady who'd helped us said.

"What do you mean, taken care of?" I asked, surprised.

She explained that Nedra had that very morning called and given her credit card number to the shop, with specific instructions that I wasn't to be told until I'd made my selection. She hadn't wanted price to influence my decision for my hair. I was overwhelmed. Such enormous generosity. Such love and kindness. I couldn't help it. I cried. So did Ray.

You remember how I told you that you need good friends to face all this? Nedra was the best friend I could have, before and especially now. She embraced me always, and with her I felt normal. Really more than normal: special. Everyone wasn't like that, of course. Another coworker became difficult, even rude. But Nedra's kindness more than made up for that. Be kind, always. You can't imagine the difference it makes.

Ray helped me cut my hair short. Short enough that the wig would comfortably slip on and stay cool, and short enough that my lost hair didn't cover my pillow each morning with long strands. Eventually, though, short enough became completely bald. The few, sparse strands of fragile hair looked so bad to me, that I wanted it all shaved off completely. Ray said it was sexy. I got used to it.

I made a whole new circle of friends. Friends that I wouldn't have set out to make, and friendship that was based on a circumstance that I couldn't have imagined for myself or cursed my worst enemy with. But friends they became nonetheless. Judy I told you about, Dr. Yanis' nurse that first introduced me to this new way of life. My chemo therapist, my radiation therapist, even the office manager who scheduled my appointments and the receptionist at radiology.

I'm sorry that I can't say the same for the doctors themselves, except for my primary physician, Suzanne Ross. They were aloof: uncommunicative and dispassionate. Dr. Passen had been direct, open, and had talked to me. But there was still detachment. My primary oncologist, Dr. Yanis, had been distant to the point of cool through all of these horrible office visits and treatments. As weakening and desolate as the long hours in chemotherapy had left me; as isolating and frightened as the radiology had made me feel, none of it made me recoil as much as the weekly visits and evaluations with Dr. Yanis. I'd gotten to the point where I was nearly physically ill with dread before each one. Ray offered that it was the way they created a buffer that saved them hurt in such a high-risk field. I didn't buy that. The nurses and therapists were as much at risk of loss as the doctors.

It got me sufficiently upset that I couldn't bear to go to Dr. Yanis for the weekly checks. I wanted to sidestep that part of the regimen altogether. It was then that I resolved to do something about it.

"You wait out here this time, okay?" I asked Ray. We'd signed in at the desk and were sitting in the waiting area.

"You sure?" he asked.

"I'm sure."

When Judy did come out for me, I got up alone and followed her to the exam room.

"Ray sitting this one out?" Judy asked jokingly as she took my blood pressure.

"I want to talk with Dr. Yanis about something, and I want to do it alone," I replied. She looked a little surprised, but assured me the doctor would be here shortly, and left me to my thoughts.

It had become desperate, the thought of coming here each week. I hated the visits, and it was mostly how Dr. Yanis related to me, or didn't. I had worked myself up to this brave mindset, and I would see it through.

Dr. Yanis began his exam with the usual referring to my chart, blood counts, vital signs and the like. "You're about done with the therapies," he said, not to me directly but as he looked at my chart. "After next week, it will be just visits here so we can check the status of your cancer."

"It's these visits I hate most," I announced. "It's these visits I don't want to make. Worse than the chemo treatment or radiation!"

Dr. Yanis looked at me, surprised. "What do you mean?"

"I mean that I don't like the way you don't relate to me, Doctor," I answered firmly. "I mean that you make me very uncomfortable. You don't talk to me, just at me, and you don't make an effort to connect." I was flushed with the effort, and a little fear about confronting him, but I'd become sufficiently unhappy that I needed to clear the air.

Dr. Yanis looked at me for some time, surprise yielding to concern, and then interest.

"I wish you'd told me you felt this way before," he finally said.

We began then to have the first meaningful exchange we'd had in the five months I'd been going to him. We began to talk, really talk, and he listened to me, really listened. I told him about what I feared most, what I didn't understand, what hurt, what questions I had, and I listed them. And he answered them; every one of them.

It was the longest visit I'd had with him, and when we'd said all there was to be said, when he'd answered all of my questions, and spent the time to make sure I understand, we stood up. And he hugged me.

"You look happy!" Ray exclaimed when I rejoined him in the waiting room.

As we walked out to the car, I shared the visit with him. I was happy. I felt maybe I was part of the process again, not just an observer. "And when we were done, he hugged me!" I exclaimed.

Be honest up front, not a patient advocate, really, but honest. And, expect it in return, that and openness. It felt like a new beginning.

Chapter Four

Snow draped over everything like a great white comforter. It made me think of my childhood and home in Newfoundland, where snow came early and stayed late and never seemed to melt off. It was strange now looking out at it from my warm living room, knowing that it would be the last winter of my life.

Ray had never been a fan of Christmas. I'm not sure why, and he never offered a reason. But over time, especially with the kids growing up, he worked hard each year at getting into the spirit. The past few years with the kids gone had put him back in the mood of not wanting it. This year, though, he was going all out. Our old, over-used and somewhat bedraggled artificial tree went in the trash, and in its stead in the front corner of the living room went a huge thick short-needled tree that looked beautiful without a single light or decoration.

The three of us sang carols as we decorated, and for the briefest time I felt almost as if I had my life back again. For the briefest time I forgot that it wouldn't be a season for me to share again.

Jeremy told us what we had expected: he and Kristina would be marrying. He'd go back to Bulgaria in June and wed her there. He had hoped we could go with him, when first they'd made their plans, but he looked up briefly and the deepest sadness flickered across his eyes. He simply said he understood that we couldn't, and we stopped singing Christmas carols, the magic gone and the truth taking over again.

Within just a few weeks of completing chemotherapy, my hair did start to grow back. It was February now, and cold, so the extra layer under my wig didn't bother me. Around the house, I went without my wig, and the short, brittle gray hair that now filled my scalp made me happy. Even my eyebrows that had thinned to almost nothing, and caused me to spend too much time trying to paint them on were growing back, thicker again.

It was during this time toward the end of treatments that our oldest son, Raymond, came to visit with his family. Though he'd been the first we told, they lived in Minnesota and with a fairly new job and three little ones, he hadn't been home yet. Now, however, was the time. I was elated to have them coming, wanting to share what remained of my health and while we were all still able to enjoy each other's company and not have to face so obviously what was lying around the corner.

His wife's family lived nearby, and they stayed with them, but spent their few days here in our house, all five of them. Three little grandchildren like steps of stairs: Lucy the oldest at five, Toby in the middle at just over two, and Tillie a baby of under a year. Matilda Rose West, actually, named I liked to think after me. For them I wore what Ray had come to call my monk's wig. It was just a ring of hair that sat around my scalp and gave the scarves I would wear a footing, making me seem not really so bald without the smooth clear skin riding up under the edges of cloth. My favorite family portrait was taken then; the little ones propped on my lap and around me.

Before they left for the long drive back to Minnesota, we got the results of the post-treatment X-rays and MRI's. While the tumor in my lung hadn't shrunk at all, it hadn't grown either. And, there were no new lesions anywhere on my spine. Dr. Yanis felt encouraged by it. It helped me feel the part I'd been playing with our son and his family. Our appointment with Dr. Passen wasn't until the week after the kids went home.

"It's encouraging that there's been no growth," Dr. Passen said, leaning forward on her chair. We sat in her office instead of the examination room in the radiology department. "But, it doesn't change the mortality."

"What do you mean, exactly?" Ray asked, tightening up.

"It would be a good idea to contact Hospice," she answered, still leaning toward us. "Give you an idea about what they offered and how they worked."

We were both stunned. We hadn't expected an announcement of remission, but we'd gotten what we thought was a clear signal of arrest.

Our hopes had been toward the years left Dr. Yanis alluded to way back when all this started. Hospice sounded like a nearly immediate end.

"Why would we need to know how Hospice works this far out?" I asked, the familiar panic starting again in my chest, the trembling returning to the base of my head.

"I think we're talking about six months here," Dr. Passen said in reply. "Maybe eight months at the most. It's a good time to get them involved."

The wind had been knocked out of me. I sat gasping for air. My cough had long since stopped, my hair had started a timid return, my treatments were finished, and Dr. Yanis had seemed encouraged. Now, this doctor was talking about my life span in terms of months. It couldn't be. There was too much unfinished business to my life.

The next few days were numb. I knew from the first, though I never shared it with Ray, that this cancer would kill me, and before either of us was accepting of the time frame. I'd had prescience, if you will. I could not see me as old, or finishing my life, my perfect life that I loved so with Ray. But, I had plans for more than six or eight months would grant me.

It meant that I would live to see Jeremy married, most likely anyway. It meant that I wouldn't live to see him get his master's degree from Yale. It meant I might not even get to see him leave for there, help him settle in, see the beginnings of his new life.

I thought desperately about my three little grandchildren who'd only just warmed my lap and what they would be and how they would grow and that I wouldn't get to have any part in their lives. I realized they probably wouldn't even remember me, they were so small. And Jeremy would have children that I'd never even see, or know their names and it washed over me like a tidal wave that the world would go on without me and I would leave my mark no more.

I looked at Ray and wondered at how he could seem so positive and strong. He often said that he'd allow no negative thoughts in our house, that people could leave those at the door or not come in. He surrounded himself with this aura of certainty, and he bathed me in it too. I worried nonetheless about what would happen to him when I was gone. We'd only been kids when we met. I couldn't imagine him doing what he needed to do by himself. Yet, there he was, pushing him and me and us toward some goal that was now beyond our reach.

*****

The next week was my weekly check-up with Dr. Yanis. I no longer dreaded my visits with him. Since we'd agreed on a new relationship, I knew I could talk with him, and him with me, and we'd listen to each other. When we related the conversation with Dr. Passen, he was upset, told us not to listen to her, and even told us not to go back. While he wouldn't contradict her prognosis directly, he seemed to give it no credence whatsoever. He did suggest we see a counselor, to help deal with all we were going through. Howard Fink was a psychologist in that very building, and he'd have his office manager make the referral and appointment.

"I don't know what to think," I sobbed when we were alone again. "I can't take this back and forth with my life."

Ray was upset too, and couldn't offer anything to comfort me. He did, though, offer a new thought in the whole thing.

"Maybe it's time we looked to other things," he quietly suggested.

"What other things," I asked, not certain where he was going with this.

"Not Mexico or something really weird," he added. "But there's lots of things going on that don't necessarily fit in the normal AMA programs."

"Like clinical trials, maybe?" I asked, feeling a little better about what he was getting at.

"Well, that too," he agreed. "I've seen a lot about those on my Internet research. But I was thinking more along the lines of some of these Wellness Centers we see. I pass one on the way to work. Or holistic practitioners. There're lots of different directions we could go."

We sat down right then and explored medical centers on the Internet, linking to their tabs that outlined their various clinical protocols. Surprisingly, there were two in progress for my non-small cell variety of lung cancer: one at Johns Hopkins and one in Texas. I wrote down contacts and phone numbers. It gave me a sense of purpose and control, something I hadn't had much of in the past half year.

That Monday morning, I watched the clock for the chance to call the UT clinical trials contact, adjusting for the different time zone. It took awhile to get through to the name I'd gotten off the Internet site, and I felt the impatience growing through me. This, I was assuring myself, might be the secret door that opens up to a gain against the clock I'd been racing. My heart skipped a beat when my wait ended with the warm voice greeting me.

"Good morning," this woman's voice said with a slight Texas twang. "How can we help you?"

I spent the next half-hour discussing my diagnosis, treatment protocol, and she gently pushed more information from me than I'd even thought to prepare to give. Fantasies are easily killed by reality, and I'd let the real aspects of where I'd been and what I'd been through stay away from my thought streams. I naively thought I'd hear encouraging news about revolutionary approaches killing non-small cell tumor growths by the legions. I'd even pictured PAC-Man snipping through my body eating every alien cell in sight.

The upshot was that since I'd already had full-blown chemo, and used some of the drugs not allowed for the trials, I didn't qualify for any of them.

"We should have asked more questions at the beginning," I said, desperately and with bitterness. "Yanis, Passen, none of them said anything about trials, or new things or ways we could go. We just went along with what they said. What they said might work. But it didn't, did it!"

It was hard to have these kinds of conversations with one of our sons back in the house, so we tried to time them for when he wasn't there. That didn't always happen, of course, and when it didn't the pain was obvious. But this time we were alone.

"Baby girl, would you have said no any where along the line to things that were offered, even knowing this?" Pain of so much conflict and doubt showed in his eyes, but he fought to stay positive and helpful.

I thought about it a good long time, and realized that he was right. What was offered had been honest in so much as anyone knew. There wouldn't have been much of a conflict. "I wish I'd known, is all," I finally said.

"Yeah, me too," Ray managed weakly. "Should we try Johns Hopkins anyway?"

It was quicker with them, smug reality haven driven my fantasy away, and it didn't take me long at all to discover I didn't qualify for what they offered. However right we felt about initial decisions, a certain regret gnawed at me, and wouldn't let completely go.

*****

33

We had our first appointment with Howard Fink that next week. I'm not sure how I felt about it. Howard, and he insisted that we call him that, was in his seventies at least. He was of the old gestalt school of psychology, was eccentric but reassuring.

"It's not easy living with this kind of sickness," he offered after a long time of general conversation. It was the first indication he even knew why we were there.

It made me cry, and I couldn't help it and I wished I could stop the tears that were coming, but I couldn't. We spent a long time then talking about it, in real terms and in real words that made me understand that he saw where we were and what we faced. We didn't learn anything new in this first meeting, but we did schedule an appointment for the next week. I left feeling ambivalent about the direction, but then I was feeling ambivalent about almost everything in my life by now.

In the second meeting with Howard, he told us about someone he'd worked with before, a retired professor from the Wright State University School of Medicine. Someone who lived in Yellow Springs and would work with people like us, in his home, for no fee, if referred. He put us in contact with Rubin Batino, and we set our first meeting for an evening of the following week.

I haven't said much in all this about my own family. They were as far away as Calgary, Alberta Canada and Freshwater, Newfoundland, and no closer. We'd visited my home every two or three years since we'd been married, with no exceptions, but had grown more apart by distance and time anyway. My parents were old world conservative, my mother a devout Catholic that had spent most of her life facing one real or imagined illness after another, and my father was stoic. Completely stoic, he never said anything about how he felt, ever. My brothers were younger and I'd always enjoyed their company growing up and as an adult through long-spaced visits. My sister and I had never gotten close like sisters are supposed to do. We'd conflicted, mostly, so she couldn't identify with anything that was going on in my life. My parents simply didn't accept it at all: I would get better, just go back to work and don't think about it.

It hurt me deeply that my parents didn't understand, or accept, what was happening to my life. I really felt like my mother didn't want the competition: she couldn't remain the sickest of the family if I was dying. It hurt deeply that my father had nothing to say, ever. So, I didn't have much support from them. It was down to Ray and the friends we'd built together, our kids, and his family that became our fortress against this horrible cancer that wouldn't let me be.

It made me think, though, more than I had since I'd gotten the terrible news last September that I needed to go home. I needed to see them, have them understand, accept my dying, and say my good-byes.

Ray and I began planning a summer trip home.

The next week we drove to Yellow Springs to meet with Rubin. The town's a throwback to the sixties, free spirited and open, with a culture that seemed locked in a time warp. Rubin's house was on a side street, nestled in trees, faded siding on a unique ranch with a garden of sculptures and ivy that nearly blocked the entrance. It didn't seem a likely place to meet someone with tools to fight the monster that had me in its clutches.

"It's kind of spooky," I said as we approached the door.

"Real hippie stuff here," Ray agreed as he rang the doorbell.

Rubin Batino was a tall man of about seventy. He had full thick gray hair and thick-rimmed glasses. He wore baggy pants and a sweater, thick and hand woven, buttoned up to his neck.

"Come in," he invited, stepping aside and motioning us in. "You must be Ray and Donna."

Rubin led us down a short, book-lined hall to a doorframe with a beaded curtain as a door. He pulled it aside, and gestured us in. It was his den, study, office or some such, with a desk, more books, a sofa, tied wall hangings, plants and floor to ceiling windows on each of the two outside walls. The kind that didn't open, were narrow, and had long since trapped enough moisture between the insulating panels so as to cloud up and be opaque.

"I try to help with visualization," Rubin was explaining after small talk. "You need to picture your own body battling the intruder," he went on. His was an approach that believed the body, if properly equipped, could manufacture its own defenses. His job was to create a mood of complete relaxation for me, help me see my own immune systems growing the army that could combat the invading cancer cells.

We spent the evening talking about pleasant memories, the kind that made me feel warm and secure, safe from things that could hurt me. He asked me to conjure up a place from my life that I could escape to, exclude the enemy, and open myself to healing from within. I recalled the high-grassed lawn up the hill behind the house that I'd grown up in. The sky blue with clouds chasing above me as I lay on my back, looking through the tree limbs that filled the small garden.

I liked the idea of the Pac-Man I'd pictured before, chomping through my blood stream, devouring ugly cells growing out of control. He had me lie back on the sofa, close my eyes, and drift back to that place. He filled my thoughts with my internal army battling the cancer. His voice was soothing, his imagery perfect, and I felt a tingle through my trunk and limbs as if an army really were moving out on the battlefield and laying waste.

It was late when we got home, and I was exhausted. Ray had been quiet for most of the drive, and I'd wondered if he was letting me rest, or was thinking about the session.

"What did you think?" I asked as we neared our neighborhood.

"Not sure," he said after a brief pause. "But then, I wasn't sure what to expect. It was certainly *alternative*," he added.

"Yeah," and I laughed in spite of my exhaustion and uncertainty. We looked at each other, and Ray smiled too. It was good to have some humor between us. It had been too long.

"I wonder what the tape will be like," I said.

"Like his session," he said. "I think I'll let you do those by yourself."

We laughed again as we turned into our driveway. Rubin had promised he'd record a tape for me to use at home, and often, to help me get my mindset in place for this new game we'd play. I wondered how well it might work. I had felt relaxed for the first time since that black day in September.

Chapter Five

A good and longtime friend of ours, Janet Neeld, had a son who was a biochemist. Bruce Neeld lived with his wife in Chillicothe, southeast of Dayton about two hours drive. Janet had us come to her house in Xenia to meet with Bruce. He wanted to help, and he was offering a special diet and supplementary regimen that would help me gain strength and develop a holistic reserve to battle my cancer from within. It was the second foray for us into alternative ways to approach my cancer.

"Your diet is really great," Bruce commented as he looked over the sheets I'd prepared and mailed to him a couple of weeks before. "Don't change a thing there."

We'd eaten healthy for the past ten years or so. I'd quit eating red meats before Ray, and eventually got him to join me. Vegetables and fruits were a big part of our diet, with chicken and fish the only meats. And, those were prepared by broiling or grilling so it kept the fat down. I was a big advocate of exercise too. We walked together between three and four miles nearly every day. They weren't casual walks, either. We managed four miles in under and hour, and many days we went to Hills and Dales Park or Sugar Creek Reserve with its woods and paths where steep hills made our heart rate soar.

"Have you been able to keep up the walking?" Bruce asked as he flipped over to the next page.

I didn't have to answer him. The look of sadness and loss that washed over me told him that I hadn't been able to manage as much for some time.

"We get short walks in, around the neighborhood," I finally responded. "Not as much as I'd like, but it tires me out so."

Bruce nodded his understanding.

After we'd gotten through all my history, including what chemotherapy I'd been on and prescription medications I was taking,

Bruce handed a sheet across the table so Ray and I could read as he talked.

"You need to beef up your vitamins and food supplements," he was saying. "It looks like you're doing a good job of keeping up on the eating, but you need more energy reserves." He reached down to a box on the floor beside him, and began lining up a row of pills, some bottles as large as a gallon milk carton. He had eight or ten bottles on the table when he finished.

Bruce went through each bottle, referring us to the sheet he'd given us, outlining what each was and what each could be expected to provide. His mother, Janet, had been taking many of these for years, through Bruce's advice, and I'd never known anyone in their sixties to be so vibrant and full of energy as she was. It was an impressive array, and each, Bruce carefully explained, was chosen in light of my particular needs and history.

Janet brought a pot of coffee to the table as I scanned the catalog that was on the table with the supplements. The price of some of them scared me, and I looked with some hesitation at Ray. He just kind of shrugged, as if to say it didn't matter.

"I'm giving you these," Bruce said. He seemed to be sensing my reservations.

I looked at him, astonished. We didn't even know Bruce before today, and here he was giving me hundreds of dollars worth of specialized supplements and vitamins. I stammered, trying to say something, but couldn't. It was the second time someone had spent a good sum of money when they didn't need to. I didn't know how to react.

"Listen," Bruce explained. "You guys have had enormous expense so far outside insurance benefits. And I know they don't cover this. I just hope you have to renew this three month supply many times over."

In addition to being energetic, Janet was one of the funniest people we knew, and we spent the afternoon laughing and enjoying their company. None of us mentioned sickness and health again. It was just a pleasant day, something too rarely found for me.

Janet, Bruce, and his wife each hugged us long and hard as we left. Both of us had our arms full as we went back to the car. Janet stood on her porch, waving at us as we pulled out onto the street.

"People amaze me," I said, crying just a little in spite of myself.

"People love you, baby girl," Ray said simply. "They want to be involved. They want to help."

It was hard for me to believe that people could love me, enough to get involved with my life with the mess it was in now. Nedra was my friend before all this, but we'd just met Bruce.

"Besides," Ray went on. "I'm guessing it was Janet that paid for that. She just didn't want you to know."

I love Janet. I always have. I tried to imagine me being that generous with people if the roles were reversed. I decided that I would.

"There's the Wellness Center I was talking about," Ray said. We'd just pulled onto the main road back to Kettering. "I'd like for us to check it out." It was on Ray's route to work, and it was closed now, but he asked if we could go together next week and see what they had to offer. I was less afraid now of checking into those things that weren't part of the mainstream medical approach.

"Sure," I agreed. "What have we got to lose?"

In spite of Dr. Yanis' instructions not to see Dr. Passen again, we felt we needed to confront her bleak prognosis. While her forthrightness had scared me, I realized she was candid, and I'd likely be seeing her again for radiation. I knew it was only a matter of time until future tests showed new tumors sprouting up somewhere else. I really did want to visualize my own army eating the cancer cells, but only as I'd listened to Rubin had I felt it might really work. It hadn't taken long for dread certainty to consume me again.

It was early March now, and we made an appointment.

"Be careful with alternative medicine practitioners," Dr. Passen said. We'd mentioned our visualization regimen, and the supplements and our plans to visit the Wellness Clinic. "They can really get in your pockets for very little offered."

I felt the sense of defeat wash over me again, but Ray had put his hand on my knee and squeezed it slightly.

"Dr. Passen," he began, "you haven't offered us much in the way of hope, have you? We don't plan to replace conventional treatments, but we're sure not going to let any stone go unturned, either."

To her credit, Dr. Passen went no further with her cautionary words. "Just keep a balance," she advised.

"Maybe she's right," I admitted when we were back in the car. "Maybe it's not such a good idea to spend a lot of money on experimental things that haven't proven anything." I don't know how many thousands of dollars this had cost us so far. I always kept the books before, but lately I hadn't been able to focus enough, and Ray had taken over that duty, along with about every other responsibility in our lives. I'd begun to worry about what would be left for him when I did die.

"Baby girl," Ray answered, stopping the car and turning to face me. "I'm not going to put a dollar value on getting you well. I don't want you to either. Okay?"

I looked at him, realizing I wasn't going to be able to change his mind. I wondered at what he thought, if he really believed I would get well again, or live past the few months Dr. Passen had again emphasized was left for us. "Okay," I agreed, not really believing it.

"Good," he said, smiling again. "Now, we check out the Wellness Clinic."

Since it was the middle of the day, and neither of us was expected back at work, we decided to go back to Xenia and check the clinic and its offerings.

There weren't many cars there, and the interior of the building didn't give a ready impression of what function it had served in the past, but it was scrubbed and clean and professional looking. The small reception office off the main hall had a desk with a white-gowned lady, who looked like a nurse. The nursing diploma on the wall behind her had the same name as the nameplate on the desk.

"How can we help you?" she asked pleasantly.

"We really don't know, for sure," Ray replied when I hesitated. "This is kind of new to us."

A look at my hair, or lack of it now that I wasn't wearing my wig full time, gave the woman a pretty clear picture of where we were.

"We deal with a lot of cancer patients," the woman ventured. "Would you like to look over our services?"

There were surprisingly few treatments offered that I would have thought might be on the list. At least I couldn't see where what was offered had to do with my needs. We already had a dietary plan and supplements regimen set out for us. And, therapy was covered by Howard and Rubin. Therapeutic massages caught my eye, however.

"What are these about?" I asked, pointing to the massage section on the brochure.

"These help you attain optimum relaxation," the woman replied. "It's more effective for your body to combat the cancer if you're relaxed. Would you like to meet with one of our therapists?"

We'd come this far, and it seemed harmless enough. Ray gave me an encouraging look, so I thought, why not.

The massage therapy room was pleasant, with subdued lighting everywhere but the desk where the therapist sat. She invited us to have a seat beside her.

"It's really quite straight forward," she said assuringly. "The sessions are about an hour long. You'll feel peaceful, almost floating when we're done. Would you like a demonstration?"

She reminded me a bit of Rubin, and Yellow Springs, with her too long hair and tie-dyed floor length dress of some gossamer fabric, richly colored and loose. But her manner was confident and reassuring. I hesitated only briefly.

"You can stay," she said to Ray. "But only if you promise to be quiet and unobtrusive."

Ray agreed and I squeezed his hand, feeling like I was reassuring him for a change. She led us across the room to a long padded table covered with a sheet and invited me to climb up on it and lay down. She lowered the lighting level some, and put a CD with tranquil music on, and asked me to roll over on my stomach.

I did drift away from there, almost but not quite to the dark fluid place where the anesthesia took me during the biopsy. I could feel sweet tingling out to my fingertips and toes as she gently rubbed my muscles and flesh, talking soothingly all the while, helping me visualize the energy she was pushing into and through my body. She conjured visions not unlike Rubin, and I lost myself in the special place she was making just for me. It was long minutes after she'd finished before I realized she was done.

"Do you think this is something you'd like to continue?" she asked.

I hadn't felt this relaxed in a very long time, the kind of relaxed that would stay with me long after I'd left. It made me feel peaceful enough that I felt I could endure what I knew was coming at the hands of the more conventional practitioners, and what my body was dealing to me.

"Yes!" I said without hesitation. "How often?" That was my only concern, how often I could enjoy this respite from my life.

"As often as you'd like," she replied. "Though I'd think once a week would be right, at least for now."

I'd enjoyed it enough that I hadn't even thought to ask how much this would cost. I knew it wouldn't be covered by our medical insurance, but it didn't seem to matter. It didn't matter to Ray either, as he encouraged me to set an appointment.

"I can drive you over here," he offered. "Maybe after lunch at home, then I can get some work in while you're here. Okay?"

And it was okay. Very okay. We scheduled an appointment for the next week, and left with me feeling more relaxed than I had in a very long time. This was our third venture into the alternative medicine field, and it felt very right.

*****

"Mom," I said into the phone. "We're planning on the end of July for a visit. Is that okay?"

"Oh, yes, honey," she answered. "That would be just fine. Kitty and Christa will be here then too. It'll be just lovely!"

Though I'd grown up in Newfoundland, and mom's voice hadn't changed much in the thirty-five years I'd been away, her strong almost Gaelic accent seemed nearly alien now. And the way she always pushed for my sister when I mentioned going home upset me. Kit was the take-charge type who always had to be in control, and in the few phone conversations we'd had since we'd told her about my cancer, she'd avoided that and seemed almost patronizing. It didn't excite me that she would be home at the same time.

"Maybe that's good," Ray said when I'd gotten off the phone and shared the conversation. "Maybe seeing Kit, and her seeing you, will help you guys get closer."

I had some unresolved issues in my life, few but some. Kit was one of them. I didn't much believe seeing her would resolve anything or heal anything. But maybe it would. Maybe there was more depth there than I'd been willing to see or admit.

My birthday was July 30, and we made the reservations for home that would put us there with that date right in the middle. We'd see how real or relevant or willing was Kit's ability to understand my life and its end.

It was my third meeting with Rubin, and he gave me the tape he'd prepared so I could try the visualization he'd created for me on my own.

"What do you want from your visit home?" he asked. Ray and I had shared our plans for two months from now.

"I'd like for my sister to understand," I answered quickly, then thought some more. "And I'd like for my father to tell me he loves me. He's never done that."

I could feel Ray tighten.

Rubin told a story about his own father, and something he'd made for him from wood and carried back on the long plane trip, looking forward to his father's reaction. Like my dad, Rubin's father was a stoic, not given to displays of emotion, and more often critical. But Rubin said his father accepted the gift graciously, and commented on its craftsmanship and beauty.

"You can be surprised by fathers who don't express themselves," Rubin said.

"You don't know Mr. Rose," Ray said. "I think it's a mistake for Donna to shoot too high. He won't give her what she wants."

"To say that he loves her?" Rubin asked. "I think he will."

"And if he doesn't," Ray countered, "and I'm certain he won't, where does that leave Donna? Why open her to that hurt?"

Ray was emotional as he said this. I knew in my heart he was right, but I wanted to believe Rubin, that he could say it and would. They discussed this at some length, Rubin and Ray, while my mind drifted through tunnels of memories and times in my life when things were extreme. Like when I'd gone off to school in St. John's, leaving home for the first time. Dad hadn't even hugged me. Further back when I'd fallen on the train tracks and split my head open, dad had been there but detached. More recently when I'd left home to marry and he hadn't held me then, or said whether or not he loved me.

Oh, I knew he did. I knew it from small ways he'd be there when I'd needed him, protecting me, picking me up, carrying me when I was too small or too tired. But I'd needed to hear him say it. And he never had. As I listened to Ray and Rubin I realized that Ray was right. He probably wouldn't. He probably couldn't.

"If it's what you want, what you need," Rubin said, "then ask for it."

"Don't expect too much," Ray said when we'd gotten back in the car. "It's not important for your dad to say that."

It was, though. It had become very important.

*****

I kept my weekly appointments with Dr. Yanis. Each one went well, with blood tests good and every apparent gauge of reckoning seeming positive. Even my work continued well. It seemed I had my life back, and while the demon dogged me, it wasn't at the forefront of every thought.

Jeremy had made his plans to fly to Bulgaria, to wed Kristina on June 8. Oh, how I ached to be there with him, to watch my baby get married, to return to the magic of the May of last year when we were completely happy. But I was grateful that I was here at all, and that I was watching his plans unfold. I could remember thinking just a few months before, at Christmas that this was something I might not live to see. But I was doing well and the time was here, and he was leaving to come home a married man.

And by the time he got home, I'd be just five weeks away from my own trip. My trip home, which, I realized with some shock, would be for the last time. I didn't like the way my cancer had taken over my life, ruled its limits, and said what couldn't be for me. Every time I let myself forget, even for a moment, it came back hard with a vengeance and let me know what was really in charge.

Over the next weeks, I saw Dr. Yanis five times, we met with Howard twice, and I'd used Rubin's tape nearly every day. I couldn't tell a difference in how I felt with Bruce's supplement program, but realized I might feel a lot worse if I weren't taking them. The massage therapist, whom I'd been seeing twice weekly this past month, had left the wellness clinic and opened her own office closer to our house. I made these visits the last of the day for me, leaving work early and then be home and relaxed by the time Ray got home from work.

With just a week to go until we left for Newfoundland, I started stopping by my favorite department stores, getting new shoes, a couple of new outfits, and things I thought I'd need for our trip. It seemed surreal to be doing so many normal things, to not be pumping toxins into my body, or being blasted with radiation, and even combing my own hair. While still gray and not nearly as soft as it had been, it was now nearly three inches long, and I delighted in brushing and combing it. The wig was still part of my work wardrobe, but around the house and sometimes even out shopping, I went with my own hair. Others might look at it and think something was wrong, but whenever I looked in the mirror, what was reflected looked encouraging, even normal.

Chapter Six

We boarded our flight in Cincinnati, connecting to the non-stop flight to St. John's, Newfoundland in Toronto. Toronto was always difficult, with long layovers, huge crowds, and we were sure that security and immigration would be really difficult in this new era of terrorist-awareness flying. We took our passports, a first for a trip to my home. That made it seem even more foreign and remote from my life.

Another first was that all we used were the carry on bags we'd bought for our European trip the year before. I wouldn't have believed I could get by for two weeks with just two small suit cases, but last year's trip proved it did work, and it made baggage claim and pickup delays a thing of the past, and customs and immigration more immediate. So, after we cleared on the Canadian side in Toronto, we made our long way through the maze of the terminals and bus connections, and got to our departing gate with over an hour to spare.

"My right foot is bothering me," I said to Ray, annoyed as we sat in the gate area. I'd taken off my new shoes and was rubbing the ball of my foot and the arch, hoping to chase away the cramp-like feeling that had begun to annoy me.

"Do you want to dig out another pair of shoes?" Ray suggested. "Hey, one of the benefits of having luggage right here."

"No," I decided. "I need to break these in anyway." The long walk through the airport complex, and so much time on my feet was, I was certain, what had caused the discomfort. "It'll be fine by the time our flight leaves. I wish my right arm didn't tingle like this, though," I added, not really thinking anything about it.

It was an uneventful flight, thank god. Flying into the Torbay airport outside of St. John's could often be frustrating, with fickle weather delaying flights, or even sometimes diverting them to Gander, Newfoundland. We had clear weather this time, and my brother Bill was at the airport to meet us. It was ten hours since we'd left home, and though I'd gotten some sleep on the flight, I was exhausted. It was dark when we left the terminal, following Bill to his car.

Bill had moved his family since I'd been home last, and instead of a suburb on the city's West End, they lived right down town in a row house. A big three story, rambling place that was semi detached from their neighbor, it turned out to be only a few blocks from the business school I'd attended right after high school. And, it was a comfortable walking distance from Memorial University, one of Bill's favorite haunts. It was a frightful old worn house, right on the busy street with no front yard, but I loved it.

Bill is an artist, both a painter and a musician. He'd started in rock groups back in the bay area of home not long after I'd left to marry Ray. He'd grown in skill and reputation, and now did solo gigs at many of the upscale clubs around St. John's historic district. His stylized guitar playing is unique, wonderful, and much sought after. His painting had begun about the time I started dating Ray. In fact, Ray had given him his first painter's textbook; one Ray had used for years. Bill cherished that book, and the interest Ray had taken in his efforts, and still had it in his library. He insisted he even referred to it now and again with help in making just the right pigment for a painting. His reputation as a painter had grown larger than that of a musician. His paintings hung in galleries all across Canada.

Bill is also quite tall, taller than our oldest son who is six-five. And Bill's wife is short. Pat is a psychologist, has her own practice, and does a lot of contract work for the government employees in the province. Between them they had three kids, two boys with the oldest one raised and gone, the second boy raised but still in St. John's and home often, and their daughter Alison, who is fourteen with blue hair and experimental jewelry and clothing styles. They're quite a family, and quite a welcome sight. I'd always been especially fond of little brother Bill, and now that I was home, he held me tight and told me how much he loved me and how worried he'd been these past months and how wonderful it was to have me home.

We spent that night with them, and most of the next day touring around the city, noticing the many changes and many of the old unchanged haunts of my youth. Bill pointed out a big old bed and breakfast that was supposed to be haunted.

"I'd love to stay there before we go home," I exclaimed, intrigued with the mystery that went with haunted house tales.

"Let's do it, then," Ray agreed. "We can come back from the bay a day earlier than we'd planned, and spend our last night there." The thought excited me.

"There's something I want to show you, Madonna," Bill said. He headed us toward Signal Hill at the gut of the big harbor for the city. When we reached the summit, he parked the car near the tower from which Marconi had sent the first wireless message in the century before the last. We followed him across the lot and up a trail.

"It's just a short distance from here," he assured me. It was sweet that he didn't want me to tire.

We stopped at the top of this small hill on the larger famous hill. Bill had told me he'd started a cairn there for me. A rock tower that he'd started with a single stone, adding to it on every visit, now stood taller than my height, and a good four feet around at the base.

"You want to add to it?" he asked, handing me a fist-sized stone.

I took the stone and stood, staring at this monument my little brother had built for me. I cried as I stretched up to put my stone on the tower.

"I pray for you, Madonna," Bill said, hugging me. "Every time I'm here I add a stone and say a prayer."

Bill had made a lot of visits, I could tell. If only prayers were really answered.

Late that afternoon, Bill took us to my other brother, Jim's house. He and Mary Theresa had been married just five years less than Ray and me, and they'd lived in the same house on the city's outskirts for the past twenty years. Their lifestyle was very different from Bill's. Both their kids were grown and gone, and their neat ranch was beautifully decorated. Jim worked in the auto supply business, and Mary Theresa was a lighting decorator. Jim always made me laugh, and was cracking jokes as soon as we hit their doorstep.

The next morning, we left for Freshwater and my folk's house, the one I'd been born in, the one dad had built. Jim drove us the two hours west and south on the Avalon Peninsula, and the rugged unspoiled beauty of the province almost surprised me, as if it were new to me. The low-lying shrubs of spruce and fir and ground cover were so green they were almost orange, and ice blue ponds dotted the landscape all along the Trans Canadian Highway.

Pulling into Freshwater, I could see that nothing had changed. Jim pulled into the parking pad beside the house, which looked freshly painted, as always. Dad hadn't been able to do such things himself for many years, but he made sure everything always looked fresh and hired most of it done.

The front door was open, and mom was sitting just inside the entrance looking out for us.

"Oh, honey," she exclaimed, "it's so good to see ye!" She stretched out her arms and I bent down and took her hug.

Dad was standing just behind her, smiling slightly and leaning on a walker.

"What's that for?" I asked, surprised. Dad was over ninety, but still took fairly long walks twice a day, swift and straight and firm. A walker was the last thing I expected him to have.

"It's your mother's," he answered. "She took a fall the other day."

"Are you alright?" I asked, turning back to her.

"Oh, I guess, child," she said. "My hip troubles me. I expect it's broken or something."

I turned and looked at Ray, and he rolled his eyes slightly. We both knew if mom's hip was broken, the walker wouldn't be of much help. It seemed to be little more than another entry in her long list of health woes.

"I never did see a doctor," mom continued. "Your father hadn't the time for me now."

I shook my head, wondering what she was thinking.

"I'll get you there tomorrow, mom, if that's what you want."

"Oh, we'll see, then, child," she said, and laughed a little.

"Ye look good, Madonna," dad said, only lightly returning my hug. "Good to see ye gettin' well."

I cringed, seeing that they still didn't believe or accept my reality. "Where's Kit," I asked, changing the subject.

"Oh, she's upstairs now, takin' herself a nap," mom answered. She stood to take her walker from dad, and pushed her way across the living room to her chair.

"Oh, hi, Aunt Madonna," Christa said, coming out of the kitchen and hugging me. "You had a nice flight, did you?"

Christa was an elegant young woman, tall and slender. Kit had raised her aware of fashions, and the willingness to spend any amount of money to achieve the perfect, stylish look. She was a good girl, though, and not as superficial as her appearance might suggest. I still couldn't get used to the idea that she was so grown up.

"Let me go get mom," she said, turning to the stairs.

We'd been able to settle in a bit, and I'd taken my wig off from the travel, with my coarse gray hair for anyone to see. Neither mom nor dad said a word. Then my sister came around the wall that separated the stairs from the living room. She rushed me, arms outstretched, and held me firmly. I was glad to see her.

Kit and I ended up in the kitchen, with cups of tea, catching us up on the latest news. She and Christa had gotten there the week before, and had plenty of opportunity to get a handle on all the local gossip. As it happened, this was a "come-home-year" for Freshwater, as well as my mom's ninetieth birthday, so ample celebrations were underway and planned. Mom's birthday wasn't for another two months, but Kitty had decided to take advantage of our mutual visits, and have a special do while we were both there. She was outlining the events she had planned for mom, and they sounded elaborate.

"Kit, how bad a fall did mom have?" I asked. "Why hasn't she seen the doctor?"

"Madonna, she's afraid of the doctors, you know," Kit answered. "She's afraid they'll put her in the hospital and she'll die there. But I don't think there's anything wrong with her. She's well able to get around."

"She's spent more time in hospitals than anyone I know," I said. "She can't be that afraid of them."

"You know how she is," Kit replied.

"I know how she is, I just don't understand why."

Dad never spoke the rest of the evening, to me or to Ray. He sat in the living room watching television until it was time to go to bed.

"What's wrong with them?" I asked Ray when we finally settled into our room late that night. "They act like nothing at all's the matter with me. Did you hear dad say I'll be fine now that I'm back to work?"

"They don't want to face it, baby girl," Ray answered.

"They're that way with everything, though," I said. It was frustrating for me, especially now. They'd never related to any problems we kids had had, growing up or as adults. And all mom could ever think about was what might be wrong with her next. "I think they're just very self-centered."

"Or scared of life, maybe," Ray said sleepily. "Just don't ask something of your dad that you know he won't give. In spite of what Rubin said."

I'd been thinking a lot about that, and had seen that as one of the most important parts of this trip. I'd come to believe it was possible because of Rubin's encouragement, but now that I was home, and all the old issues were right there, I had to agree with Ray. It bothered me more now to think about how dad would react if I asked him for affirmation, but I still felt it was something I needed badly enough to ask for it.

Mom's birthday party was to be the next week, just two days before my birthday. This week there were lots of visiting opportunities because of the "come-home-year" celebration going on in the small town. It was an event someone staged every five or ten years to encourage those who had moved away, and there were many, to come home en masse and see one another and pump some vitality into the quiet, aging and decaying town of Freshwater.

Tonight, our second in Freshwater, was a big outdoor dance just down the street in the church and community center parking lot. I wish my hair were its bright shiny self, but I pulled my wig over my head and carefully combed it to look as much like mine as I could. I wanted to look my best seeing these old friends.

It was hard to believe so many people had come home for this, though many may well have been on personal missions like mine, though none were quite like mine. Anyway, the large asphalt area was overflowing with people milling around the performance stage where various local and provincial bands were playing. There were two or three beer tents, and there were two bars open in the community center, which was full as well. Probably more people were here from away this evening than generally lived in the town.

I'd rested most of the day, visiting with Kit and mom between naps, saving my energy for this evening. But, after no time at all, it seemed, my right foot began bothering me; to the point where I needed to sit down.

"Do you mind if we go inside for awhile?" I asked Ray. We'd been meeting friends from my childhood and cousins from far away and local. None of them made any reference to my cancer, though I imagine most of them knew. They all hugged me and told me how great I looked.

"Sure, baby girl," Ray answered. "Are you feeling alright?"

"I just need to sit for awhile," I replied. "My foot's bothering me again. Plus, the band is getting to me."

Ray took my arm and steered me through the crowds and into the community center. We looked for a table and found two open chairs at one across the main room.

"Can I get you something to drink?" Ray asked.

I hadn't had any alcohol for quite some time, and thought maybe a cocktail would make me feel better, or at least take my mind off of my cramping foot. "How about a gin and tonic?"

When Ray got back with our drinks, a couple had sat down across from us, and the man was smoking a cigarette, flicking his ashes into an empty beer bottle. There was a large "No Smoking" sign right behind them, and several more throughout the room. Ray started to lean across the table and I grabbed his arm.

"Don't say anything, honey," I cautioned him, leaning near to his ear. "They're a pretty rough bunch and I don't want anything starting."

"Christ, baby, you're fighting lung cancer and this idiot smokes in a no smoking area? I don't think so," Ray countered. He was getting upset.

"Maybe you could say something at the office," I suggested. The couple, the man especially, was well known in the area as being fighters and bullies. I didn't want Ray getting into a fight with him, and he was getting angry enough that he might have. Thankfully, Ray took the suggestion and left the room for the front desk and the hall manager.

There were more people smoking in the room than just the people across from me, and the smoke was beginning to make a cloud in the room. I knew we should leave anyway when Ray came back and helped me out of the chair.

"You're not going to believe this," Ray said as he hurried me out of the building. "The manager said they weren't going to enforce the no smoking rule tonight. I guess we're stuck outdoors with no seats."

It was getting late anyway, nearly ten, and the trip fatigue and my cramping foot were taking their toll.

"Why don't we go on home," I said. "I'm getting pretty tired anyway."

"Are you okay to walk, or should I go get your dad's car?" Ray asked.

It was only a half mile or so, and I didn't want to stand waiting while Ray brought the car back. I thought the walk might even help ease the cramping. "Let's walk, if you promise to go easy on me," I replied.

Ray laughed, took my hand, and we started up the hill toward home, the crowd noise and lights faded behind us, but the music dominated the cool night air right up to the front door.

Mom's birthday celebration started with a Mass, and the small sanctuary was filled, with family and friends from quite a ways off sharing in the service. Mom enjoyed her special status, and sitting on the front pew, the priest directing all his attention and comments to her. Dad sat beside her, stiff and formal and us kids were in the pew just behind them, with cousins and other family behind us. Mom and dad had the distinction of being the oldest folks in this small outport town, so there were lots of locals paying their respects. Neither mom nor dad seem to acknowledge any of them, though.

The priest talked about loving families with close ties, deep and rich histories, and how like those great stories my family was. It wasn't a family that I identified with, but he'd built his opinions on what mom had told him, and I was sure Kit had helped nourish that image.

Jim's daughter, Cathy, is an accomplished musician, and from the choir loft at the back of the church offered beautiful flute melodies during the service. I watched as people bent their heads in earnest prayer and found that I wasn't able to join with them. Their God had deserted me, and I felt no desire to offer prayers just to be ignored.

The Mass was followed by a reception in the community hall that last week had hosted the town's party. This time, the no smoking policy was firmly in place, and I welcomed the chance to sit and visit with family and friends. Kit had done all the planning for this, down to the catered lunch that filled two tables along the side of the room. In front, the dais with a microphone was draped behind with a large banner wishing mom a happy birthday.

Cyril Reilly, a childhood friend of my oldest brother Bernard who wasn't there, was the emcee, and made the program of music, readings and reminiscences entertaining. The next door neighbors, the Mulloleys, growing up had a house full of kids and the now grown daughters, who'd long ago moved away, sang tributes to mom. Both of the boys, John and Gerard, had died as fairly young men. I'd actually dated John some, but

Gerard, Gerardie I'd called him when we were little, had been a closer friend and a coworker at the town's bank years ago.

Cathy, with her flute, and her boyfriend, a guitarist, provided music for the gathering between programs on the stage. My brother Bill had brought his guitar, and soon he was doing extraordinary stylization, and we all sat rapt, caught up in the beautiful melodies.

It was a nice day, relaxed and fun, and aside from the cramping in my foot and the increasingly annoying tingling in my right arm, I was free from thoughts of my illness and the future that would be stolen from me.

"A lot of your friends told me how much they admired you," Ray told me when we were back at the house.

"Really?" I was surprised at this. "In what way?"

"You didn't seem at all bitter to them," he answered. "They couldn't get over your easy way and ready smile."

It wasn't something I thought consciously about, so to hear this came as a surprise. I'd often wondered how people kept going, once they'd gotten a death sentence: how they'd found the strength and reserve to be normal. I'd never realized that normal was a relative thing. Though it might not be normal to others, a good day for me without pain or great fatigue, was wonderful.

Chapter Seven

My father had been born on Red Island. On a day without the coast's normally dense fog, its red silhouette was visible on the eastern horizon from Castle Hill, above Freshwater. It was a big part of local lore, and mostly deserted since the government-forced resettlement program of the mid nineteen sixties. Ray's first novel, *The Price of Men's Lives,* had a substantial reference to it as a fishing ground for the men in the bay who made their living from the sea. I'd been there, years ago before I'd met Ray, but he'd never been there. He was nearly done writing his newest novel about the island and the disruption of lives, and sorely regretted that all his references had come from research on the Internet and family albums with faded photos rather than a first-hand visit.

Mary Theresa's brother owned a 32-foot trawler; the hull designed and built for fishing, that he'd fashioned into a pleasure boat. Ray wanted badly to make the trip, and had called to find out about a charter.

"I'd really like it if you would go along," Ray pleaded.

Water and boats were things I'd grown up fearing. The cemetery by the bay was filled with grave markers listing captains lost at sea. He was making a strong case for my revisiting my roots, and my resolve was giving way.

"It's important to you, isn't it," I said. There was an almost urgency in his pleadings.

"It would make the place more alive with you there," Ray said. "I think I could understand it better, feel it more, if you were with me."

I knew what he meant, and I had to admit that it would be good for my own peace of mind, this close to the end of my life, to feel and smell and taste the place so near to where I'd grown up, but so far from my life.

"I'll go," I finally said, smiling.

Ray hugged me tight. "I love you, baby girl. Thanks."

We went to the wharf in Dunville, just two miles outside of Freshwater on the way back to the TCH, where the boat was tied up. My brother Jim had decided to join us, but had been especially hard to wake up this early in the morning. Kit's daughter, Christa, had decided she wanted to go as well. Like Ray, she'd never been there, but had heard about it all her life. Kit hadn't wanted to get up, though, so stayed behind.

Fog was burning off by the time we stepped aboard the trawler, and the early morning sky promised to give us a nice clear day. Ray was completely in his element as he climbed onto the boat, timing his step to the rocking from the waves. He'd always loved boats and the sea, as much as I'd always hated them. It was the only real conflict in our lives. He was adamant about boating, and had finally won out. He'd built a twenty-two foot sailboat some years before, and though I had never looked forward to it, I ended up going out with him most times. Now, with a fair sized boat on the ocean, he was in heaven. I got on board, quickly found a seat in the cabin, and hoped the voyage would be over soon.

The *Joseph Smallwood,* a liner-sized ferry that sailed between Nova Scotia and Newfoundland, and was named after the province's founding premiere, cut through the large expanse of water some distance out from our bow. It looked noble out there, sailing between Red Island and us, and for a moment I could understand the exhilaration Ray seemed to feel when on boats. All this was my heritage, I reminded myself, that I'd so willingly given up thirty-five years before to start my life with Ray far inland.

The dark, solid red landscape of the island began to develop features. White dots clustered near a rock outcropping became houses, and soon the bleached, weathered pilings of wharves took on distinct lines contrasting with the rock and water of the harbor's shoreline.

It was eerie, really, pulling into the spacious natural harbor on Red Island's western shore. Nothing seemed to have change from my last visit here some forty years before, except that now two or three of the houses were lived in again, and a very few fishing boats were tied along the wharves. None of the settlement's churches still stood, and the small family run stores were gone. I gazed out through the boat's large window at the dock growing nearer and wondered how such life cycles of whole communities would go on after I died. In spite of myself, I quietly cried.

"Come with me," Ray invited, reaching down from the dock to where I stood on the boat's aft deck.

"I'm not up to much exploring," I said, reaching for his hand and allowing him to help me up the ladder boards nailed between two pilings. I stepped over the rail and onto the planked surface.

"I'm going to walk around the harbor, see the houses and stage-heads," Ray said. "Do you want to stay here or go with me?"

There was another, smaller boat, tied to the wharf, and a fisherman was loading his cargo of fish from his hold into large tubs on the dock with a big net hung in a sling from a davit. Two of the island's full time residents, a man and woman, ran the fish collecting station, and were helping the fisherman.

"I think I'll just visit with those folks," I said, not wanting the exertion of walking the winding path over rocks and streamlets that connected this side of the harbor with the houses on the other side.

"I'll go with you, Uncle Ray," Christa called out as she pulled herself up the ladder and onto the dock.

The two of them disappeared around the storage shack of the small fish collection business at the end of the dock, heading for the path to the little cluster of houses. I watched as they reappeared down by a small waterfall feeding into the harbor, step over some boulders, and make their way through the brambles that lined the way. Oh, how I would miss seeing Ray so excited with discoveries. How I would miss sharing his exuberance and special talent of telling his stories of Newfoundland to others back home. He was more in his element here than I was.

The couple, in their mid forties, had been here four years. They were one of three families that called Red Island home. Since the fishing industry largely collapsed from over fishing some ten years before, processing plants that had dotted Newfoundland's shore were gone. They were replaced with way stations that held in refrigeration the few fish still caught until weekly visits by large factory ships that took the area's catch to plants on the mainland. These people were pioneers of sorts, giving up a conventional life among people in real communities. They got their energy from the isolation, and peace and quiet, of the largely deserted harbor town.

They lived across the harbor, and a beautiful, big, and very new looking longliner was tied to the wharf and stage-head by their house. *Red Island Rose* was painted in beautiful script across her transom, white letters in sharp contrast to her gleaming navy blue hull. The man had built it, with the help of his wife, and they shared a photo album that chronicled its construction.

"Don't you worry about needing doctors?" I asked. I couldn't imagine being so far from help if it was needed.

"Not much them folks can do for ye," the woman said. "If it's your time, then you're done for."

Her comment burned through me like a shot. Most of my life for the past ten months had been at the hands of doctors and nurses and therapists seeking to find a cure for my cancer, or a release for me. Yet the simplicity of her observation was right there, and entirely true. There wasn't much those folks could do for me, in the end, and I questioned the wisdom of continuing the fight they wanted me to wage. I even briefly considered how idyllic it would be to escape to this place for what time was left to me.

"It's just amazing, how these people live," Ray exclaimed as we pulled out of the harbor. His enthusiasm was obvious.

"It is," I agreed. I didn't share the part of the conversation I'd had about doctors, but I did tell Ray about the boat the couple had built.

"It's beautiful," Ray said wistfully, standing in the door frame at the cabin's rear, gazing back at the island, which was becoming a red cliff on the horizon again. "I admire them all." It was obvious he could live here, at least for a time. Over the years, especially during visits home, he'd scan the paper's classifieds, seeing what jobs might be open. He wanted to live in Newfoundland as much as I didn't want to live here. Though the urge seemed to pass after we'd gotten home for a few weeks, it always attacked him while visiting. It was something else for me to wonder about, whether or not I'd been right in objecting to such a life change.

The captain put the boat in idle some two miles out of the harbor, and took fishing rods and tackle out to the aft deck. "We'll have some nerve twitchin' fresh fish for our lunch," he said, passing by me. "You fishin' with us?"

I didn't really feel like leaving the warm comfort of the cabin. Even though it was now the start of August, the sea breezes off Newfoundland's coast had a cold snap to them. Ray and Christa, however, eagerly took some gear and followed the captain to the stern.

Over the years, Ray had frequently gone out with the fishing boats, working hard at hauling up nets heavily laden with large cod. He would delight in bringing home a bucket of cod tongues that my dad would carefully wrap in small bags for the freezer. It was a delicacy that few but the fishermen could enjoy. But, since the fishing on that scale had ended, Ray hadn't been able to crew. I watched him carefully now as he tossed his line out into the ocean. It wasn't the kind of fishing he was used to, but he was on a boat, out at sea, and trying to pull fish out of the water. I wondered if this was the life he would choose for himself after I was gone. My eyes moistened as I considered his having a life after me, and not being able to care for him and share it all.

The boat's stove was soon on, and the crackling of fish in the iron skillet joined with the aroma, filling the cabin. It was good, and though I didn't have much of an appetite, I enjoyed the few strips of freshly cooked fish Ray offered to me.

When the boat was underway again, Ray joined me on the bench seat of the small dinette. There was a large window just over the table, and we gazed out at the green ocean and gray-blue sky. An iceberg drifted past the bow, some miles away.

"It is beautiful," I admitted. I'd never really seen the beauty that Ray had always seen. Maybe growing up with it made me take it for granted. This was the first time in many years that I'd gone out on a boat in this part of the world just for the fun of it.

"Oh, it is," Ray agreed. "And exciting too." He put his hand on my leg and leaned over and kissed my cheek. "Thanks for coming along."

I was glad I did, for myself and for him. I wanted to share what experiences were left to us, and I knew all of this was Ray's great love. I didn't return his kiss, but stared back out the window. I was so tired, and feeling cheated. I didn't want him to see the sadness in my eyes.

"Are you okay?" he asked.

He was always checking with me about how I felt, whether or not I was tired, or if I was having a good time. I managed a weak nod, but couldn't return his gaze. He gently patted my leg.

"I'm sorry, baby girl," was all he said, and left me to my thoughts.

"Look, Aunt Madonna!" Christa called out. "We're being chased!"

I turned and looked out the open back door of the cabin, where she had perched herself by the rail. Behind the boat, jumping and dancing through the boat's wake, a family of porpoises leaped out of the water, arching briefly in the sunlight, then crashing back into the water. It was a delightful sight. They chased along behind us for some time, before breaking off and swimming their own way.

As we approached the harbor for the towns of Placentia, Jerseyside, Dunville and Freshwater, the drawbridge raised ahead of us, the small amount of traffic stopping on either side. On nice, sunny days like this, the people always stepped out of their cars to lean over the road's railings to get a better view of the ships coming through. I'd done that several times over the years, but it was a new thing to be on the boat looking up at the people, wondering what they thought. I had a pang of understanding for Ray's intense love of all this. I wished I'd worked harder at sharing it with him over the years, and was grateful I'd decided to come along, however much I sensed what loss lay ahead for me.

"Mom, where's Kit?" I asked when we got back to the house. We hadn't spent any time at all together since the first night. She was always on the go somewhere, visiting friends or, I suspected, hiding out.

"She went out to Long Harbour," mom answered. That was her husband, Harold's, boyhood home. No one from his family still lived there. In fact, few people still lived there at all. "She took dad's car and just left an hour ago."

It was nearly an hour drive from Freshwater, so she wouldn't be back before supper. "What's out there for her to do, mom?" I couldn't help feeling resentful. She seemed to be working hard at avoiding me, and this was too obvious a dodge.

"Visiting, I suppose, child," mom answered, not turning away from the television.

Hurt, I turned and went up the stairs. The day had been tiring, and I needed a nap, though I would have happily given that up to spend time with my sister. Instead of sleeping, I lay on the bed, staring at the ceiling, and thinking about my trip home so far. Most of what I'd seen good about it was what Ray so loved: the ocean, boats, wharves, scenery, and the sense of small community bustling about with what seemed important in their lives. I'd loved our time in St. John's with brothers Bill and Jim and their families. And it was nice to have seen and talked with old friends from my childhood at the community center.

But, the time with my family had been very hard. I'd never understood my parents, how they felt or what they thought. Dad was so detached that I considered not asking him for what I most wanted: needed. And Kit. As kids we'd never been close, she being older always considering me a pest. But now, grown up and me dying, I would have hoped she could see it for what it was, and make some effort to bond with me. Instead, she avoided me. I slept some, but the thoughts of my life made it restless.

It was Monday now, and we were flying home on Wednesday. Ray had made reservations for Tuesday night at the haunted bed and breakfast, and I looked forward to the adventure.

"We're leaving tomorrow, you know," I told mom as we sat in the kitchen drinking tea and having small cakes. Mug-ups they call them in Newfoundland. I missed the tradition living in the states, and especially enjoyed it now.

"Yes, child," mom replied. "I'll miss ye so 'til next time ye comes up."

Kit was standing at the sink, pretending not to pay any attention to our conversation.

I couldn't argue with her anymore, and knew I wouldn't make her understand, so I said nothing.

"We could spend this evening together," I said to Kit.

"That would be nice," she agreed. "I can't spend any time today. Some of the crowd over at the vocational school are meeting me for lunch. Maybe when I get back?"

"Sure," I said. "That's fine."

Ray came in just as Kit was leaving. He'd been mowing the yard for dad. Dad was really funny about that. He'd never say anything, or ask for the help, but he'd drag the mower out of the shed behind the house and leave it sitting there, so Ray would always take the hint and mow. Dad didn't do that when Harold visited, or my brothers for that matter. Only Ray. And Ray never shirked the obvious duty, nor was he ever thanked.

"What do you want to do today, sweetie?" he asked as he washed his hands at the sink. "Any thing you missed?"

"Let's just take a drive," I said. "Out to Fox Harbour or something." Fox Harbour was a nothing little sort of community, maybe ten or fifteen miles from Freshwater. I'd walked out there as a teen, going to some dance or party or something. I hadn't been there in a number of years.

"Ye can use dad's car if ye like," mom offered.

"Fox Harbour it is, then," Ray said. "Maybe we can go on out to where the Atlantic Charter was signed from there. According to the brochure I got at the Visitor's Bureau in St. John's, there's supposed to be a new park out there."

It was nice, just the two of us, driving out the road past the beautiful scenery. Rock cliffs, wild stunted spruce trees, and ice blue ponds painted the landscape as far as the eye could see. Just the gravel road and the power and telephone lines reminded you that you weren't completely removed from civilization.

It was exhilarating, being home and seeing all this beauty I'd mostly taken for granted. Maybe that I knew I'd never see it again made me drink it all in, hungrily.

Fox Harbour was unchanged, except the small bar and grill at the entry to the town was now closed. The single road split beyond that, one way leading off to the right where what was, for the most part, the town. To the left passed some houses, wharves and stage-heads, the little clapboard shacks on the shore side of the docks that served the fishing boats as storage. We swung to the right, past the school, post office and small store, heading out toward the new park Ray had mentioned.

I'd never been here before, even though it was only half an hour from where I'd grown up. The view from the small hill by the water's edge was spectacular. Giant rocks grew up out of the water, stabbing the sky. Breakers ripped through them, splashing the ocean on the gravel beach. An enormous navy anchor, painted shiny black, centered the circular monument by the wood's edge, and a brass plaque told the history of the famous meeting between Roosevelt, Churchill and Stalin more than a half a century before.

We walked along the water's edge, holding hands and not talking, just enjoying our company and the wonderful, bright day. However much I wanted not to be, I was growing tired.

"I wanted to spend some time with Kit tonight," I said, breaking the quiet. "Maybe we should head back." It was late afternoon, and I thought I might even take a nap before spending the evening saying goodbye to my only sister.

It was almost dark when we pulled into Freshwater.

"Kit and Christa are gone off," mom said. "I think to the ferry terminal or something."

"Will she be back soon?" I asked, surprised that she had taken this last evening to go off somewhere. "What's at the ferry terminal anyway?"

"Oh, the gift shop, I suppose," mom answered. "And Mary Theresa's sister run's that ye know. Maybe to visit with her."

Disappointed and tired and with no appetite, I decided to take my much needed nap. My foot cramped so bad, and the tingling in my right arm and hand had started to become a numbness of sorts.

"Wake me when she comes home, will you?" I asked Ray.

"Sure, baby girl," he said. "Get some rest now."

I climbed into bed, the room completely dark, only for the porch light reflected on the window, painting the lace curtain pattern across the opposite wall. I fell asleep at once.

I felt Ray move on the bed, and stirred awake. It hadn't seemed like any time at all.

"Is Kit home?" I asked, starting to push up out of the bed.

"No," he answered simply.

"What time is it?" I asked, settling back on my pillow.

"It's after ten," he answered. "I think it's time we went to bed for the night."

I couldn't believe it. Our last night, and Kit knew we hadn't spent any time together. Tonight was supposed to be for us to visit. I fell asleep crying a little. Ray held me and rocked me and tried to reassure me. I was exhausted, more mentally than physically. What a disappointment, I remember thinking before dreams became my world.

Chapter Eight

"You can't leave today," Kit protested. "We haven't had any time together." She was sitting in the kitchen when I'd walked in.

"We've got reservations in St. John's for tonight," I replied. I wasn't feeling very friendly, and a lot deserted.

"Cancel them," she said, almost like an order. "I'm leaving tomorrow, too, and this is the last chance we've got."

Where were you last night, I wanted to ask. Why have you ignored me for the past two weeks, I wanted to know. But I knew I wouldn't win with Kit, and was too tired to protest.

"Kit wants us to stay tonight," I told Ray back in the bedroom.

"Are you sure?" he asked, surprised. "You were so looking forward to the adventure in the haunted manse."

I was, but I asked him if he'd cancel our reservations anyway. He didn't argue or try to talk me out of it. He just hugged me and assured me that if that's what I wanted, that's what we'd do.

I went back down to the kitchen, and found mom sitting by herself.

"Where's Kit?" I asked.

"Gone off to Placentia," mom answered. "She'll be back soon, I'm sure."

I spent the day instead looking through old family albums, at us when we were kids, together, free from worry and pain and illness. I shared stories with Ray I'd never told him, and got some joy from the memories.

"We need to get packed," Ray finally said. "It's almost four, and we haven't done anything yet. We leave for St. John's early, you know."

He was right, and we went up to the room to organize for our trip home.

Kit came home as we were finishing supper.

"Come up and we'll have our time now while I pack," Kit said, again making it sound like an order. I followed her up the stairs and into the room she and Christa had been sharing.

"You've ignored me the whole time I've been home," I said. "Why?"

"Don't be silly," Kit answered, pulling clothes from the bureau drawer and stacking them on her bed. Christa's suitcases were already packed and lined up by the door.

"I'm not being silly," I protested. "You waited until we were leaving to say two words to me. Now I missed my bed and breakfast adventure." I was hurt, and didn't mind that it showed in my protest.

"You can do that next time," Kit said off handedly.

"You don't get it, do you, Kit," I said.

"What is it I'm not getting, then," Kit said, turning to face me for the first time.

"There won't be a next time," I replied. I just looked back at her.

"You don't know that," she stammered. "You might be back lot's of times." She shifted her weight and folded her arms in front of her. "Besides, I don't want to leave here with just you and Ray in the house with mom and dad."

"What are you talking about?" I asked, confused.

"Christa told me what Ray said to her the other night. Cathy heard it too. About mom and dad being geriatrics and how sad it was they were stuck in the house with them."

I couldn't understand what she was talking about, until I remembered the past week one night when everyone was gone but mom and dad in bed, and Ray and I watching television and the two girls in the dining room. Cathy and Christa had been working on the memory album for mom's birthday party, and Ray had joked to them about them being stuck with us old geriatrics while the town partied.

"Ray was talking about us, Kit. Him and me," I said, realizing the confusion. "Besides, he wouldn't use that word for mom and dad, even if that is what they are."

Kit was getting angry, and I didn't know why.

"I don't know what it is you want from them," she said, ignoring my explanation. "Calling them names isn't nice, and I get the feeling you want something and don't care how you get it."

I was incredulous. Kit was attacking me, and for what?

"Kit, you don't want to talk with me, you don't want to share time with me, and you don't want to admit the truth about me," I said, just as forcefully as Kit.

"I don't want to end the visit this way," Kit said, shifting gears. "It may be awhile before we see each other again.

I gave up. Whatever demon possessed Kit had her firmly in its grasp. She had always been overly protective of mom and dad, sure that she was the only one who could care for them. But now she was being completely irrational. I turned and left the room. Left Kit to pack by herself. I went back to our room and cried myself to sleep.

I didn't hear Ray come to bed, and the next morning was surprised when he gently woke me.

"Kit's leaving," he said. It was barely light outside. He'd been up for awhile, helping to pack the car with Kit and Christa's luggage, filling every space in the trunk and back seat. They never traveled lightly.

Kit was crying as she hugged me, apparently forgetting last night completely. Or, more likely, pretending no unpleasantness had occurred. "Be nice to mom and dad," she said. "They're old."

Old, maybe, I thought, but they'd outlive me. I hugged her back, reluctantly, and said nothing.

We were leaving in just two hours, and I had to get showered and dressed and pack what remained of our things.

It was soon our time to leave, and Bill waited patiently for me while Ray packed our two suitcases into his car.

"My foot hurts really bad this morning," I told Ray as we readied to say our good-byes.

"Leave those shoes here, baby girl," he said. "They're too cheap to fit right, and that may be the problem. Wear something else home. We'll get a good pair of comfortable shoes this week. I promise."

I agreed, and left the shoes I'd bought for the trip in the entry vestibule, putting on a pair of older sandals instead.

It was time now for us to leave, and while earlier I'd thought of little else but mending fences with Kit, which didn't work out, and asking dad to say he loved me, I hadn't thought about it for the past few days. Now we stood on the porch saying goodbye.

"Call now when ye gets home," mom said, crying and hugging me. "I misses ye so when you're gone." She told me she loved me, held me tight, and told me to get well.

I turned to dad and put my arms around his neck.

"I love you dad," I said, hugging him. "I need you to tell me you love me too. Will you say that, please?"

Dad lightly returned the hug, but said nothing. I lingered there a bit, hoping he'd say it, but he didn't and finally Ray said it was time to go. We left, mom and me in tears. My tears were because the one thing I needed most was not given to me. I left my childhood home for the last time, and felt a greater loss than I dreamed I could suffer.

"Please, baby girl," Ray asked softly. "Don't let this upset you. You know the old man loves you in his way. He just can't say it, for whatever reason."

"He knew I needed to hear it," I insisted through my tears. I was sobbing and couldn't stop. We were nearly to the TCH and the final leg of the drive to St. John's and the airport. Bill sat quietly behind the wheel, checking on me with quick glances in the rear view mirror. I had centered my whole emotional strength on just two things for this trip, and neither had worked out. And, both were such simple things.

"Why is he like that?" I asked, gaining some breath between crying jags. "Why can't he just tell me?"

The pain in Ray's eyes was real, and deep. He did his best to comfort me, but I could see that he was as unsettled as I was, and getting angry too.

"I wish I knew, baby girl," he finally answered softly. "I wish I knew."

I knew that he had wished Rubin had said nothing. I knew that he saw it as an impossible expectation. He'd shared his reservations several times after each visit with Rubin, and cautioned me not to put myself at risk. But, I had, and now I was devastated.

"Madonna," Bill said softly as he held me. He wanted to stretch the time to our departure through the security gate. "We all love you, all of us. Dad too." He looked down at me with such tenderness and understanding in his eyes, though they were clouded with sadness and concern. "Please, believe that. I don't know why mom and dad are like they are, but they do love us all, you especially. Mom never stops talking about you."

"Dad doesn't, though," I said. I was still crying some, still deeply and freshly wounded by dad's rejection.

"Dad doesn't talk about anything," was all Bill could respond with. It was true, and we both knew it. Only I'd wanted and needed this so badly, I had fooled myself into thinking he would finally make an exception; finally show an emotion.

It was all I could talk about on the plane. It bothered Ray a lot, and I could see that he wanted me to put it aside, to forget it. But, he never asked me to. He only listened patiently and gave me the reassurances he could.

The Toronto connection was even harder going back. The old comfortable sandals didn't seem to make any difference to my right foot, which was cramping horribly now. Ray had to pull both our suitcases through the airport because the tingling and numbness in my right hand had gotten worse. And dad's seeming detachment from my life and illness burned through my chest, and my head throbbed. It seemed like countless hours until we were finally on the plane headed for home.

"I don't want to talk with Kit, if she calls," I said in the car as Ray drove us home from the airport. I'd been mostly quiet since we'd boarded the last plane, and completely quiet in the car. But this was something I'd decided during our last conversation before we'd left. This was something that I needed to do, to put myself back in control, or at least a sense of it. This may be something I wanted to do to retaliate, and since I couldn't reach dad, I could strike out at Kit. She'd make her pain or anger known to mom, and dad would hear about it. I wondered some if I was being unreasonable, or even childish, but it was the only strong course I felt I could take, to say nothing of my decreased energy reserves and the need to focus on me.

"Are you sure?" he asked, surprised by the determination in my voice.

"I'm sure," I answered simply.

Ray didn't say anything, but I knew he thought I was making a mistake.

Dr. Yanis examined me carefully, checking my right eye, hand and foot.

"I don't understand it," he finally admitted. "I'm going to order a brain scan, though."

Ray had called his office early the next morning from our return, telling Judy, my nurse, the worrisome symptoms. He was in another room as he'd made the call, and thought I was out of hearing. He'd sounded worried and stressed and had insisted Dr. Yanis see me that same day. Now he was sitting pensively when I returned to the waiting area.

"What did he say?" Ray asked as we walked toward the elevator.

"Let me just hold your arm, okay?" I asked, wanting him to slow down, wanting to balance myself on him. "We need to go to the testing clinic in Centerville," I said as we stepped out of the elevator. "Dr. Yanis ordered brain scans, and they're expecting us."

Ray's faced washed white, but he said nothing as he helped me into the car. Just since yesterday I was having problems balancing myself, putting weight on my foot. It couldn't be just trip fatigue, jet lag. But, that's what I kept telling myself it was.

I stayed in bed the next day, too tired to work, extending my vacation by a day. Ray had gone into work, reluctantly leaving me alone, and making me promise I'd call him as soon as I heard anything from the doctor's office about my brain scan tests. All the symptoms seemed a little bit better as I lay on the bed, staring at the ceiling, unable to really sleep. Seemed better, but were they really. My body seemed too ready to fool me, and my mind seemed more than willing to play along.

"The scan appears normal," Judy said. She'd called late in the afternoon. The test results were sent to Dr. Yanis and he'd screened them immediately. "Dr. Yanis would like to see you next week. See if things are getting any better, but for now, it seems there's no brain complications."

I should have felt relieved, but the worrisome quirks that had developed hadn't gone away, and I felt lost not knowing what was going on.

"That's wonderful!" Ray exclaimed when I called him. He was due to leave the office any time, but I'd promised to call. "We'll figure out what's wrong, but having a clean scan is really good news." He was so upbeat, so relieved, that I didn't want to share my private fears. It was easier and more hopeful to bask in his good feelings.

His positive energy continued all that week and into the next, the only thing bringing him down was my depression over my father's rejection of my request that he simply tell me what he felt. That, and

Kit's unforgivable treatment of me. Dad's rejection was the hardest, though. I could cut Kit out of my life, which was what I planned to do. But dad, that was harder, and more hurtful.

"Maybe we should visit with Howard again," Ray suggested one evening during dinner, the week after our return. "He might give you a grounding of sorts for this." I hadn't been able to quit talking with Ray about it, and though he'd ceased to write it off to dad's insecurities or peculiarities, it clearly had been bothering him. "It's hurting you too badly not to do something."

So we did go to Howard, and I told him how disappointing my family had been on this closure trip, especially with dad.

"It's hard for you to be this sick, isn't it," Howard said, the question more of a statement. It was the same question he'd asked during our first visit, but then I was too new at it all to fully understand. Then I was dealing with just my sickness, and hadn't been hurt by other people's reactions. Now I knew just how hard it really was.

"It is hard," I admitted, and cried in spite of my best efforts. "It's so very hard."

Ray squeezed my hand firmly, and I turned to him to see tears running down his face. I knew it was as hard for him, maybe harder.

"It's hard for your dad too," Howard continued. "He wants to protect himself."

I understood what he was saying, but I felt so deserted, that I couldn't really accept it. Ray was so angry with dad that he wouldn't allow the defense, although he kept from saying too much to me. I could feel his hurt and anger.

"We have to take love as it's offered, sometimes," Howard went on. "Not like we want it. I'm sure you're loved by him."

I wished I could be as sure. The session didn't really help me feel any better, and it didn't seem to help Ray either. It would take some work, this accepting people's strange ways of dealing with me, dealing with illness, dealing with inevitable death, and I didn't know if I even had the energy.

Jeremy and Chrissie were due to come back from the short-term job he'd gotten with a forestry company in South Carolina. We'd missed their wedding, and I had watched, more than a dozen times, the videotape he'd brought back. It always left me feeling empty, shortchanged.

"I want to have a wedding reception," I told Ray one day, just a week before they were expected home. I'd planned it in my mind since we'd come back from Newfoundland, unsure as to how long I had and how I'd feel. I wanted to do it before they moved east for Jeremy's work to begin on his master's studies at Yale in September.

"That's a great idea," Ray replied.

We immediately began making plans, deciding on who would cater it, when it would be, who we'd invite. I wanted it as a surprise for them, so we didn't say a word until they got home, just a few days before the date we'd set.

"Oh, that sounds exciting," Chrissie said happily when we shared the plans. They'd only gotten home the day before, a Wednesday, and the invitations had said it was for that Saturday. It was a complete surprise to them both.

Jeremy and Ray made the trips to Dorothy Lane Market on Thursday, getting the final details ironed out for party trays, cake décor, and beverages to be picked up Saturday morning. Chrissie helped me get the house cleaned and ready. It was exhausting, but I was happy and excited. Thirty people, family and friends, would invade our home in just two days, and share with us our joy with Jeremy's wife, however delayed it was.

It was wonderful having the house full of people for a happy occasion. We hadn't entertained at all for the past year, and this made me feel alive and vibrant. People were gracious, loving and supportive, and for a few hours that wonderful day, I felt alive and well. Well enough that that evening, after every one had left and the four of us were alone, I wanted to help plan their move in two weeks to Connecticut.

I led Jeremy and Chrissie around the house, and especially the kitchen, picking things they liked to supplement what they had and would need to set up housekeeping. The table and chairs on our screened in porch would be their dining furniture. Glassware and cookware that I seldom used would make their kitchen complete, and oriental rugs that were laid out over our wall-to-wall carpeting would cover the floors in the apartment Jeremy had arranged.

Ray had picked up a U-Haul trailer, towing it with the Jeep, and Jeremy and he had spent the day before packing it full, then jamming the overflow into their small car and our back seat. Now, we were driving through Pennsylvania, following Jeremy and Chrissie, helping them start the next phase of their lives. It was exciting, and I worked hard at ignoring the near numbness that had taken over most of my right side. It was a progression I hadn't shared with Ray.

We spent the night near Wilkes-Barre, and arrived in New Haven early the next afternoon, Labor Day weekend. Their flat was on the third floor, with steep, narrow steps that I knew I could manage only once or twice. Ray saw my fatigue, and worried that I'd overdo it.

"Why don't you sit here on the step," he suggested after we'd come down from the tour through the apartment. "You can keep an eye on the trailer while we're lugging this stuff up there."

It made sense, because the neighborhood didn't look like a super safe one. It wasn't a ghetto or anything, but it was inner city, and very worn.

"Okay," I agreed, gratefully, and took up a station by the door where I could see the cars and trailer. I was exhausted, my foot ached, and my right hand was tingling and numb. It was a welcome relief. I tried to focus on my job, pretend it was important and distracting, but I couldn't shake the awful fear that was growing and consuming me.

Jeremy had arranged for a friend from his Peace Corps days, who lived nearby, to help with the move. But Ray was anxious to start, and a young man from a first floor apartment appeared, and offered to help. They had most of the trailer unloaded by the time Jeremy's friend showed up.

We spent the night on their futon, the windows open and the nearby highway traffic keeping us mostly awake. It was a warm place, and though stacked with boxes, held promise for a nice home for them over the next two years. I lay there, listening to Ray's restless sleep, and cried for the loss that awaited me. Cried for knowing that I wouldn't be here in two years to see him get this diploma, or share in his victories along the way. Cried for knowing that this would likely be the last time I would share space with this wonderful young son of mine. All of my fears and bitterness danced before me that night. All of my disappointments, current and future, paralyzed me, and my whole body felt like my right side.

We left that Labor Day morning, Monday, and started our drive back. I wanted to grieve for this last goodbye, but I felt so sick and so tired, that all I could feel was numb, and a wanting to be home and rest.

Chapter Nine

I went back to work, at least as much as I could. Partial days, mostly. I started early enough, but ran out of steam by mid-afternoon. My boss was wonderful about it, and I was getting the more important parts of my bookkeeping job done. It bothered me to settle for less than the perfection I'd always sought, but I was learning to make a lot of compromises in my life.

It was early September as I struggled with day-to-day living, trying to make my job work, dealing with my hurt over family shortcomings, and adapting to the increasing limitations the right side failings had presented to me. I'd begun to notice a numbness in the right side of my face, and this was the fourth or fifth day for that. I hadn't said anything to Ray, or called Dr. Yanis, or anyone else.

I was at work on a Wednesday morning, and had booted my computer. The display came on the screen, and I squinted, trying to focus on the characters that lit the screen. Instead, I saw blurry objects that had no definition or meaning, and what I did see seemed to roll on the screen like a television tube about to burn out. I struggled with the keys, and my vision, but things were out of whack, and I couldn't make sense of them.

"Ray," I cried into the phone. "I can't see my computer screen, and I can't make my fingers work the keyboard!" I was beside myself, panicked, not knowing what was going on, not understanding this loss of senses.

"Just sit there, baby girl," Ray tried to reassure me. "I'll be there in half an hour. We'll get you home and rested."

The calm in his voice was forced, and at odds with the feeling that rose in me, tore through me, and left me breathless.

"I can drive home," I said, unsure that I really could. I wanted at least this much control in my life.

"Baby, I don't think you should," he replied, almost urgently. "Let me come get you."

"No," I insisted. I wanted this control. Needed it. "I'll see you at home."

And that was it. I stood from my desk, panic overtaking me, everything a shade of gray and blurred in my vision, and made it to the front of the store, where Nedra sat at her station. I could barely trust myself to stop and tell her I was leaving. My mind raced, my pulse slammed my heartbeat through my veins, and I trembled with fear as I pushed open the door and made my way across the parking lot.

Ray was home, waiting anxiously in the garage when I pulled in. I was near hysterics, and when the car stopped, I shut off the ignition and collapsed against the wheel, setting the horn blaring. He was there, pulling the door open, reaching across me to pull me up, ashen and panicked, he helped me from the car.

"Baby girl," he nearly wailed. "What can I do?"

It struck me that he didn't offer condolences, didn't say things would be alright, didn't bring an upbeat mood to this. He was in stark terror, the same as I felt, and it scared me to my soul.

We were in Dr. Yanis's office the next morning, and Ray did all the talking this time. I was too frightened to say anything. I knew in my heart what was going wrong. I'd known when the brain scans came back clear that something had been missed. I felt so out of control now that I didn't want to participate at all.

I didn't hear much of what they said, but Ray's tone was more frightened and rushed than it had ever been. Dr. Yanis had Judy make a call, and the next thing I knew Ray was pushing me across the parking lot in a wheelchair to the hospital elevator for a MRI.

"Why didn't they do this before, if it's more sensitive?" I asked, confused by the introduction of this new test. I'd known from what was going on with me that the scans hadn't revealed the truth, but I hadn't realized there was something better.

"I don't know," Ray answered. There was no anger in his voice, or panic, but there was a deep dread.

Ray sat down across from me at our kitchen table. He was shaken, his eyes reflecting fear, but he tried to seem calm. I was terrified, but certain of what he was going to say. Dr. Yanis's office had called him at work with the MRI results, and he'd come straight home to tell me.

"There are cell clusters, baby girl," he said. He stopped, checking his emotions and taking a breath. "They're on the left side of your brain, and some close to the stem."

I took it in, and waited a long while to respond. It was a deadening sensation that took me over now. It was a certainty. I had seen the cancer growing up my spine from that tiny lesion on my back, almost from the day they told me it was there. I'd tried to hide from it, tried to fool myself it wasn't going to be. But, I'd known the truth, and here it was.

"Are they sure it's cancer?" I asked, weakly. I knew the answer.

"Oh, baby," Ray said, and leaned into me pulling me tight to him, and trembling.

And so I did go back to Dr. Passen. Ray told me that Dr. Yanis had explained that chemotherapy wouldn't work in the brain environment on this cancer; that radiation was the only course. Only it wasn't Dr. Passen this time; it was another doctor in her office, a young man whose name I can't even remember.

I had my first dose of radiation that same day. It was in the same radiology treatment area that I'd been to before, but this time they made a clear plastic mask that form-fitted my face, and put their marks on it. The therapist didn't seem so upbeat as the one before, and I wasn't as in tune with what they were doing. It was all in a fog.

The next treatment was for the next day, and there were sixteen treatments in all, scheduled every day for two and a half weeks. This second time Ray parked in the emergency room parking area so we could walk straight down the hall to the treatment area. This second time I could still walk, holding Ray's arm for balance, by being careful with my steps and thinking about each one.

The third day I wasn't sure I could walk that far. My balance was shaky at best, and my right leg wouldn't go where I wanted it to, even with thinking very hard about it.

"Honey, I'm not sure I can make it walking on my own," I said to Ray as he helped me out of the car. "Can you get something to help me?" I tried very hard not to sound helpless. I didn't even try not to sound scared. Somehow I was beyond that now. I wasn't accepting, but I was resigned.

Ray got a walker at the entrance, and it helped me balance better than just his arm. We got down the hall and to the treatment.

On the fourth day and the fourth treatment, Ray brought a wheelchair out to the car, and helped me get from one seat to the other.

On the fifth day, I told the therapist I wanted to see the doctor again.

"Will I regain use of my leg and arm?" I asked the young doctor, sitting across from me in my wheelchair and Ray in a chair beside me. "Will my vision come back?"

"We can't repair the damage that's done," he answered clearly. "But maybe I can adjust the angle of dosage. I can't increase it, or risk further brain damage. But, maybe we can slow this down."

My right arm was mostly limp by now, and I had trouble focusing on the doctor's face.

"Slow it down?" Ray asked.

"We can't eliminate the cell clusters," the doctor explained. "We can buy time."

"How much time?" I asked, rejoining the conversation.

"Maybe as much as six months," came the answer.

Just six months, I repeated to myself. All that I've been through, and now this for just six months. It was a six months I didn't care to live, I suddenly decided, not like this.

"It's a quality of life issue now," I said distantly, detached. I turned to look at Ray.

"Will you take me home?" I asked.

Ray's face was tortured. He knew what I'd decided, and he was biting down on the inside of his mouth, fighting to avoid saying what I knew he wanted to say. Silently, he stood and took the wheelchair handles, and pushed me toward the door.

"Tomorrow's treatment will be adjusted," the doctor said.

"I won't be back tomorrow," I said simply, without looking back at him. I couldn't believe the strength of my voice: or my resolve.

My hand trembled as I held the phone, waiting for Ryan, my boss, to take my call. I dreaded this. As long as I'd been able to work, I felt I had some control, and some hope. Now, I was calling to give it up. He'd been so fair to me that I couldn't pretend with him, or myself, that I'd ever be back, ever able to do my job again.

"If there's anything we can do, please tell us," Ryan said. "I mean it. Anything."

Ray was in the kitchen, watching me carefully, as I hung up the phone.

"I'm taking family leave at the end of this week," he said matter-of-factly. "I'm calling Hospice tomorrow and find out what they can do to help us."

"You can't give up your job," I protested. "Not even for a little while."

"It's already done," he replied. "I spoke with personnel this morning. I need to be here now, to take care of you."

"It wasn't supposed to be like this," I protested, and began crying. I couldn't believe, in spite of my acceptance, that all the plans for our future, all our years together, loving and sharing and looking forward to growing old together, were now over. Future dreams would never be ours.

Ray knelt beside my chair and slipped his arms around my hips. He looked up at me with such sadness and resignation, and love.

"I love you," he said. "There's no more important thing in all the world for me now."

He buried his face in my lap, and sat still for so very long. I stroked his hair, looked down at him there, and wondered, with great fear, what would happen to him.

Monday was Ray's first day of family leave, and the hospice counselor was there just after lunch, interviewing us, referring to the medical charts that had been forwarded to them by Dr. Yanis, and assessing what we needed.

"I'll be Donna's primary care taker," Ray said as we talked with the counselor.

"We have home visitation nurses that will bathe her, when it comes to that, and help you with care," she replied. "It's too much for you to try to do alone."

"No one bathes her or cares for her but me," he insisted. "We'll need a nurse to check on her, but care is my job."

"I'll assign a nurse," she replied after considering Ray's resolve. "A registered nurse that keeps us up on pain management and reporting. What do you need for now?"

Ray had been a Hospital Corpsman in the Navy, and had served with the Marines in Vietnam. He was skilled in health care, and assessing needs. He always doctored the kids when they'd hurt themselves, and had always known what was best to do.

"Donna's having trouble getting around," he answered. "A walker would be helpful. Can we have that?"

"Certainly," the counselor replied. "Anything else?"

"It's been hard for her to shower, and lift herself from the toilet," he said. "Can you provide appliances to help with that?"

The counselor promised a walker, a toilet seat elevator, and a shower seat. "When these aren't enough, you'll let us know?" she asked.

"I'll let you know," Ray promised.

This was the Ray that I'd always known; always loved. He was confident and in charge. He'd harnessed some power that gave him the strength that had eluded me. He was practical and firm, resolute and determined. It gave me a sense of peace and comfort to see this new affirmation replacing the recent fragile persona that had so nearly collapsed him just the week before.

It was September sixteenth, and the Hospice counselor had left, leaving us a schedule and contact name and number for the nurse that would be helping Ray. It was early afternoon, and we still had much of the day ahead of us. Summer warmth still held the days, and leaves had only started turning toward the brilliant colors that I so loved.

"What would you like to do with this day, love?" Ray asked, seeming to flirt just a little.

"Could we go for a drive?" I asked. "I'd like to see the trees turning."

We drove to Fort Ancient, about an hour from home, where fall colors promised excitement, and the weekday promised solitude. We'd gone before, when I was healthy, in the fall and walked trails and meadows at the base of the Indian Mounds. Then, it was always weekends, and small children ran around us and past us on Saturday outings with their parents. Today, though, it was only ours. And I couldn't walk past the pavement where we'd parked.

"Let's grab that picnic table," Ray said before I could feel the exhaustion. "We can see everything from here."

He helped me through the small grassy area, and sat beside me on the bench. It was wonderfully quiet and peaceful, and golden leaves had replaced green ones, and red tints started painting across others.

"Who'll tell you what this looks like next fall?" I asked, idly scanning across the thick woods. Ray was color blind, and I'd always oohed and aahed over autumn trees, telling him in detail what each tree looked like. All he could ever see was the same hue that had clothed the trees in summer. Even the brown leaves of late fall never seemed to look different to him.

"I won't look at trees next fall," Ray said haltingly.

"You will, honey," I protested.

"I won't, you know," he said turning to me. "I'll never like fall again. Fall was yours, and not for me, alone."

I welled up with a feeling of such sadness and desolation. Was he sharing with me what his life would be like from now on? Was he saying he wouldn't want to live any more?

"You've got to promise me you'll still look at the trees," I said to him. "Will you promise you'll look for me?"

Ray looked at me, trying very hard to hide his sadness.

"Let's enjoy this fall, together," he countered. "Let's just enjoy now."

He looked away from me, and in spite of his efforts to hide it, I saw the tear on his cheek. I couldn't help it. It made me cry.

That first week entirely together was a wonderful week, and a frightening week. We were together constantly. Ray cooked breakfast, took me to lunch, made dinner, and we spent our evenings watching old videotapes of our trips to my home, when the kids were young, and Key West at Christmas, and Christmas at home, and Easter at Uncle Joe's farm. And we laughed that in every video everyone was eating. Food seemed like the central part of our lives. I'd never noticed it before.

It was frightening because before the week was over, Ray had told the nurse on her first visit that we needed a wheelchair. I just couldn't push myself with the walker any more. It was frightening because the shower chair wasn't enough, and Ray had taken to showering with me, washing my bare scalp, where radiation had killed my hair for the final time, while standing in front of me, and kneeling to help me wash my body.

It was a reassuring week too, when Ray came back from the mailbox with a card from his work. I sat in the wheelchair at the kitchen table, now rearranged to accommodate this new need, while he opened the card and read it. I turned to look up at his silence, and he was crying.

"What is it, honey?" I asked, concerned with his tears and sadness. But it wasn't sadness at all.

"Look at this," he said, and handed the card to me.

I opened it, and it was filled with gift certificates from Take-Out Taxi, good for all my favorite restaurants. There was a sheet with menus for each. The certificates were for twenty-five dollars each, and there was a thick pad of them. I counted them out, and there was six hundred dollars worth of them. The card was signed by nearly everyone I'd ever met at Ray's work, or heard him talk about. Both sides of the card, and the back, were filled with signatures. I cried too. I had never seen such generosity.

"We don't need to worry about going out now," Ray said, a smile replacing the tears. "And, you can invite friends over, and show off even."

It was a delightful surprise, and I began thinking about who we could invite to share this good fortune.

"You've got to work with me, baby girl," Ray was saying. He was trying to lift me out of our bed to guide me to the bathroom.

"I can't," I pleaded. "I can't make my leg work." It was so frustrating not to be able to even stand up with help.

"Just this once," Ray promised, struggling to nearly drag me across the bedroom. "I'll call Hospice for a portable potty to go by the bed. You won't have to make it so far then."

I worried for Ray, that he would damage his back, which had been a problem since he'd broken it years ago. I didn't want to have to make him do this.

"I'm sorry," I said as he eased me down on the toilet. "I'm so sorry."

"It's alright, baby," he replied. "We'll be fine."

His strength amazed me, physically and emotionally. He never hesitated to respond to any need I had, even anticipating some. He never complained or never got mad at me; no matter how much trouble I was becoming.

Ray's brother Larry, and his wife Frannie, came to dinner that week. I'd asked Ray to call them, and order from Jay's Seafood Restaurant using some of the gift coupons. We hadn't been able to visit them for awhile, and Frannie was like a sister to me. More of a sister than my own. And she always claimed that I was her sister. We enjoyed a great meal of grilled salmon. We laughed and caught up on family news. Ray cleaned up after, and Frannie and I stayed at the kitchen table with some coffee while Ray and Larry went out on the back porch to have a drink. It was easier with my wheelchair not to try to move around the house any more than I needed.

"How are you doing, sweetie. Really." Frannie asked when we were alone.

"Oh, Frannie, I'm so frightened," I answered, not concealing my tears.

"I'm so sorry, my love," Frannie said patiently. "I wish I could take all this away for you."

"I know," I said. "Thanks for being here for me."

Frannie reached across the corner of the table and gave me a hug. "Is there anything we can do to help Ray? Maybe he needs a break."

"He wouldn't take it if he could, Frannie," I said, leaning back in my wheelchair. Just reaching into her hug exhausted me. "He does everything, and doesn't ever seem to get tired. I'm so worried about him. Now, and after I'm gone."

Tears streamed down Frannie's face, but she smiled through them, great love in her eyes.

"He's my hero, Frannie," I said. "He's been so strong and patient and caring with me. He is my angel in all of this. I couldn't do this without him."

"We did good with our hubbies," she agreed. "We got the best of the West's."

It was a line we'd both used often in our silly girl talk when we'd complain about how our men sometimes got on our nerves. We both agreed many times in the past, and especially now, that we wouldn't consider trading them.

They left early, concerned with how tired I got.

"Call me, sweetie, if you need to talk," Frannie said leaning down to kiss my cheek. "Call me for anything."

Chapter Ten

It was the second week of October now, and Ray had been giving me bed baths for the past four or five days. I could no longer balance on the seat in the shower, and he hadn't been able to lift my dead weight to get me there. It was hard for him to bend down and wash me. The strain on his back forced him to stop frequently and stretch, give himself a break.

"This isn't working too well, is it," I said as he bent down to finish drying me. "Maybe we should call Hospice and have me admitted there."

"No, baby girl, we'll manage," he answered, lifting me to put a clean nightshirt on me. He'd bought three bright colored cotton nightshirts that pulled easily over my head. It's all I'd worn for the past week.

"You can't keep this up," I protested. "Besides, we both know I haven't got that much time left, and I can't die here at home."

I hadn't actually said I was going to die before, at least not to Ray. It wasn't as hard to admit as I expected it would be.

"This is the only place you'll die, baby girl," he insisted. "It's your home. I won't let you die anywhere else."

It seemed easier for him to say this than I would have expected. We both were more at ease with this pending reality than I would have imagined, especially since we'd never said it point blank to each other before.

"But our home is sacred," I argued.

"And that's exactly why this is where you'll be," he said with finality. I knew he wanted me here, more for me than for him.

"We can get a hospital bed from Hospice," he said. "We can take the couch out of the family room and put it there."

The thought pleased me. It was my favorite room in the house. I loved seeing the fire crackle in the fireplace. The television was there, and it was in the center of things. I wouldn't feel left out imprisoned in a bed in the back of the house.

"Where will you sleep," I asked as Ray struggled to lift me and turn me into my wheelchair.

"Right here," he said. "We can get one of those baby monitors so I can hear you, if you need anything."

"Are you sure you want to do this?" I asked.

"I'm sure."

Things were so changed with us sleeping apart. Ray spent his days in the family room with me. He kept the blind open beside the hospital bed so I could see out. It was a long summer, and though it was into October, not many leaves had fallen. They still held their color, and I could see the neighbor's yard across the street and enjoy the bright colors.

Our oldest son Raymond flew into Dayton, with our granddaughter Lucy. It was delightful to see them. I asked Ray to move me into the recliner chair at the head of the bed before he left for the airport. I wanted to put my best face on for them. They lived so far away, and even though I knew Raymond understood I was dying, I wanted him, and especially Lucy, to see me as normal as possible.

"Mom, it's so good to see you," Raymond said, leaning down and hugging me, kissing my cheek. "I think about you all the time." He pulled back and as he did, his cheek pushed my head cover aside, and I could see that he was unsettled by my hair having fallen out again. We hadn't told him that.

"Hairs too much fuss for your dad, and for me," I said smiling. I wanted him at ease. "I want Lucy on my lap."

Lucy was five, and a little shy with me. I knew she sensed things were terribly wrong. But, she climbed up on my lap and gave me a hug.

"Nana, can you see?" she asked as she sat there.

"If I want to," I answered. Things were so out of focus for me that it was easier and less disconcerting if I kept my eyes closed. I opened them to look at her. "See?"

"I don't think you can see too good," she said looking up at me.

"Good enough, sweetie," I replied, and squeezed her. It was funny how honest and open she was.

They stayed for three days. Raymond had brought his video camera with him, and wanted to interview me.

"I want this for the kids, mom," he said. "So they won't ever forget their nana."

It was hard, but I held back the tears that were so ready to pour out. He asked me questions about me and my childhood, about Ray's and my early years together, and about he and Jeremy growing up. It was strange, but I had trouble recalling things, even recent things. He tried to correct me a couple of times, but finally gave it up and let me answer however I wanted. What I wanted was to get it right, but things just weren't there for me.

Their last night, Lucy insisted on sleeping in the family room with me, so Ray got a sleeping bag out of the attic, and made her bed on the floor.

"I love you, nana," Lucy said sleepily in the darkened room.

"I love you too, little sweetness," I answered, and soon heard her steady breathing of sleep. I wondered if I'd ever get to see her again.

The chaplain from Hospice visited for the first time that week. She was a tiny woman, sweet and patient, and spent her visit just finding out how I felt about things. In fact, her name was Patience, and I couldn't help thinking how right that was.

I was raised Catholic, but had moved away from the church over the years. Ray was a Methodist, but took catechism and converted when the kids were very young, so it wasn't just him that made me grow alienated to my religion. I'd never believed it all, and in the past year felt so deserted by any god that I was angry toward the church and religion. My mother was devout, and sent me prayer cards and amulets almost every day.

"Would you like a priest?" Patience asked. "If you'd feel more comfortable with that, we can arrange it."

I liked her right off, could talk to her, and she was more a good listener than anything. I was perfectly happy with her visits.

"Will you come back if I say no to a priest?" I asked.

"As often as you'd like," she answered.

It was a comforting visit, and I could hear her and Ray talking in hushed tones in the kitchen before she left.

"What was that about?" I asked when he came back to the room.

"I'm sorry, baby girl," he responded. "I didn't mean to shut you out. Patience just wanted to know how I was doing, and if there was anything I needed."

I don't know if that was the truth or not, but he seemed sincere, and I knew he was well intended. I was afraid of things that I might not know, and didn't want to be left out of any discussion about me.

"If you say so," I teased. "I do need a kiss, though."

Ray bent down, slipped his arm around my neck, and kissed me gently on the lips.

"Could you lie down with me for a bit?" I asked. I so missed our intimacy.

He sat up on the bed, and lay down beside me, putting his head on my shoulder.

"Do you want to make love, baby?" he asked timidly. He was so afraid of hurting me, but his offer made me so happy.

"I want to," I admitted. "But I can't. I'm so numb and things aren't working right." It was horrible to admit I couldn't, but his closeness felt so good. "Just lay here and hold me."

We both fell asleep, and took a long nap in each other's arms.

Over the next several days, every catch in my breath at night would bring Ray running down the hall from the bedroom.

"I'm having trouble getting enough air," I finally admitted. I felt terrible that he couldn't get a night's rest, and his days were so busy waiting on me.

"I'll call Hospice in the morning," he said, comforting me. "We'll get oxygen brought in. That should help you breathe."

And so I learned to breathe through a hose. It made it easier, though. The thing that worried me most was that Jeremy was driving down from Connecticut and would be here in two days. What would he think about this, I wondered? But I'm blessed that both my sons are caring, loving men who can be great diplomats.

"Mom, it's so wonderful to see you," Jeremy said, bending over the bed and holding me, kissing my cheeks. I couldn't manage the recliner for his visit, and it bothered me, but he put me at ease.

Jeremy sat on the bed, and told me all about his life with Chrissie in New Haven. Their apartment was all straightened up and very much lived in. Chrissie was doing well with her new job, which was what kept her from making this trip with him. His studies were going well, and he loved his new life.

I hungrily held onto every word, asking so many questions, and living as best I could his life with him. Jeremy is so smart, and we're so proud of him. How I wished I could be there when he graduates.

The two days of his visit were wonderful, and when he left, I cried. Cried for seeing him leave, and crying for never seeing him again. We neither one said that, but we both knew it. I made him promise to look after his father for me. I'd asked the same of Raymond, and I needed to know that they would fulfill their promise.

"Don't worry, mom," Jeremy said. "We'll look after dad. I promise."

He left and I felt empty. I'd said my goodbye to him and his brother, and the finality of it left me drained. How I wished I could have such closure with my own family, my sister and my father.

My parents called while Jeremy was home, and spoke with him briefly. As they talked with me, both of them said they hoped I'd get well, and dad even suggested if I got back to work, I'd feel better. Laying here in the hospital bed, with oxygen feeding my lungs, and relying on Ray for bed baths, my right side mostly paralyzed, and an increasing problem with swallowing, their naiveté made me angry, and made me cry. Why couldn't they accept my fate, and support me in what was inevitable.

Kit had called once since I'd been bed ridden, and Ray had fielded that call, telling her I didn't want to talk with her. She'd been angry and rude with him, but he held his ground. I'd insisted on it. Since then, her husband Harold had called twice, checking on me through Ray. I was conflicted with my decision not to talk with her, but I was determined she would understand my hurt and alienation. Still, when Nedra visited, I blamed Kit for the lack of contact.

"Even my own sister won't come see me," I complained. I know I was seeing it only from my point, and maybe not with a clear thought process. But it was how I felt. When Nedra left, Ray saw her out then returned to my bed.

"You know, baby girl, if you asked, Kit would be here in just days," he said, sitting on the edge of my bed and holding my hand.

It was hard for me to imagine that a simple request would bridge a life long gap, and heal the wounds of our words just over two months before.

"Do you really think so?" I asked, considering the likelihood of her responding that way.

"I do. I'm certain of it," he replied. "Would you like me to call her?"

I considered this, agonizing over whether or not it was worth the risk of rejection. Whether or not it could make a difference. There were only two unresolved issues in my life: Kit and dad. If I could close this chasm between myself and Kit, it would be a huge weight off of me. I knew my need from dad would never be satisfied, so this was especially important.

"Would you?" I asked.

Ray got up and went straight to his study. He was back in ten minutes.

"Kit wasn't home," he started. "But, I talked with Harold. He said this was the call that Kit had been praying for. He said she'd call this evening."

"Oh, Madonna," Kit was crying into the phone. Ray had brought it to me without a word. "I'll be there by Monday, I promise!"

It was a Friday now, and her friend with Air Canada would help her make special arrangements. She said she'd call Ray the next day with flight arrival information.

"Madonna, I love you so," Kit said before hanging up. "I'm so sorry about what happened."

It left me in tears. They were bittersweet tears of joy that my sister wanted to see me that badly, and sorrow that we'd wasted so much of our lives and opportunities to get it right. She was sincere and anxious. Monday would be a benchmark day for me.

It was Sunday, I think. The blind was open beside my bed, and the shadows across the lawn made me think it was late afternoon. I'd been thinking, or dreaming maybe, about what it would be like when Kit got there. Earlier, I'd heard Ray talking with someone on the back porch. It was only his voice, so I guess he was on the phone with someone. I hadn't been able to make out the words, but his voice was agitated.

It was a strange day, with me mostly sleeping and Ray quietly sitting beside my bed. He liked to sit there with his hand wrapped around mine. The quiet was interrupted with the phone ringing. Ray slid his hand off of mine, and reached for the phone. Right beside me, I could hear his words clearly.

"Hello."

There was a slight pause.

"Yes, Mr. Rose," Ray said.

Another pause.

"She's right here, and I think she's awake."

I felt him shift his stance, move closer to me.

"She probably can't say much, Mr. Rose," Ray said then. "But she can hear you, I think."

Ray bent toward me.

"It's your dad, baby girl. He wants to say something to you. Okay?"

I nodded, and Ray put the phone against my ear.

"Madonna?" dad asked.

It was hard, but I managed a weak "Yes, dad, it's Madonna."

His voice hesitated, but he finally spoke.

"I loves ye, Madonna," he said. "I've always loved ye."

I couldn't speak. Tears welled up and streamed down my cheeks, the new dampness pasting the phone to my ear. My lip quivered, and I started crying. I couldn't believe what I'd heard. I couldn't believe that my father had actually told me that he loved me. I was so completely happy.

"I wants ye to be well," he said finally when I'd said nothing. "I knows ye can't, but I wants it anyway."

I managed a whisper.

"I love you too, dad. Thank you. Goodbye."

Ray lifted the phone from my ear.

"Goodbye, Mr. Rose," he said. "I'm glad you called."

Dad had told me he loved me, and my sister was coming to see me. There was nothing unresolved in my life.

The neighbors behind us, around the corner really, were separated, but the woman, Marcia, knew about my cancer, and had offered to come a couple of times a week and read to me. She was a nurse, and it gave Ray comfort to be able to leave me now and then to run errands and know that I was in good hands.

I enjoyed her company, and the freedom it gave Ray to get a little time for himself. I couldn't really enjoy her reading efforts. I couldn't follow the story line, and more often than not would drift off to sleep while she read. Still, she came and sat with me and read to me.

As it happened, Kit's flight was due in during one of her promised visits, so Marcia kept me company while Ray drove to the airport. It was especially important to him that someone qualified, like Marcia, could be with me. I had problems in the last few days holding my bladder until Ray could get to me. And I found it harder and harder to swallow all the pills I was on now. Most of them were pain medications, and Ray had started grinding them up with a mortar, and mixing them with apple juice that he fed me through a straw. He knew Marcia could do this, and respond to any accidents I might have in the bed, while he was gone.

I could hear the door open, and sensed that it was Ray and Kit. My hearing seemed extra perceptive now that I was loosing other senses. I hadn't opened my eyes in days, didn't even know if I could, but the hearing made up for it. I knew when she came breathlessly into the family room. She dropped her suitcase and came straight to my bed, where she leaned down and wrapped her arms around me and cried. She held me so tight, and I was too weak to hug back hard, but I did manage to bring my left arm up around her neck.

"Oh, Madonna," she said weeping. "My little baby sister Madonna." It was all she could manage, but she held me tight and long, our tears mixing on my cheeks and staining my pillow.

I was helpless now, and I no longer fought it. I couldn't even feed myself, but Ray and Kit helped me eat, helped me get out of the bed to use the portable pot that was beside it, and kept me bathed and in fresh nightshirts. Ray even showed Kit how he changed my bed sheets while rolling me first to one side, then the other. Ray had been so precise and so careful and considerate in doing all of this over the past days and weeks, but it was new to Kit. She was amazed at the care I took.

I could hear them talking in the kitchen.

"My return is for Sunday," Kit said. "I'll stay 'til then if you want. If you want me to leave earlier, just tell me.."

"Kit," Ray replied to her, "it's good for you to be here with Donna. She needs this, you know. I won't ask you to leave early."

I knew that Ray wasn't comfortable with Kit, and that he had been angry with her for the way she treated me when we were home in August, but he wanted me to have the time I needed with her to set things straight. I was glad they were getting along.

"Don't you need more help?" Kit was asking him. "I don't know how you manage by yourself."

"I'm not by myself," he told her. "Hospice has been a great help. You'll meet the nurse in charge tomorrow. They've been a godsend."

The rest of their conversation faded out. I tried to concentrate on what they said, but I was so tired, I just let myself drift off.

"I gotta go," I realized I was moaning before I was even completely awake. Ray was there instantly, and Kit was right behind him. It was the second night for her, and the first she realized that I needed care at night.

Ray struggled to get me out of the bed and turned to sit on the potty.

"Can you manage?" Kit asked, surprised with the effort it took, and wanting to help.

"I don't know," Ray answered her. "I've got to."

It took the both of them to get me back to bed, and the strain on Ray was obvious. I was dead weight now, and I hated it. But try as I might, I couldn't help at all. Kit hovered, concerned, and stayed with me for a while after Ray had gone to bed.

"Oh, Madonna," she said quietly, almost to herself. "I wish that there was something I could do."

It was increasingly difficult for me to say what I wanted. The thoughts were there, but I couldn't coordinate my mind and my tongue. I looked at her and carefully framed my reply.

"I wish so too, Kitty," I managed in a near whisper. "Help, Ray. Please."

Things were changing so fast, that I knew I couldn't live much longer. Today had been hard for me to take the food Kit and Ray had tried to get me to eat. I wanted to eat, but my tongue kept pushing the food back out. I wanted to swallow, but the reflex just wasn't there. My mind moved easily between all this and my past and something I didn't recognize or understand. I wanted to ask Ray what it was, or Kit, but I couldn't verbalize my questions.

Kit was napping, and Ray was at the head of my bed, adjusting the oxygen supply. I felt like I was slipping away, spending more time with my mind confronting this new unknown sensation and stimulation than with where I was or what was happening to me. I suddenly had the clearest vision of my being gone from this life, and Ray alone to go on, and start a new life. I wanted him to, but I didn't want to be forgotten. It was a fear that had started to haunt me these past weeks.

I focused my mind on my thoughts and fears and needs, and turned my head as much as I could toward Ray.

"Don't ever forget me," I asked quietly, just above a whisper. I wanted to shout it, but couldn't.

"How could I ever forget you, baby girl," he responded. "You're everything to me. How could I not think of you every day of my life."

I wanted him to hold me, saying this. I wanted him to say more. I wanted him to confess his fears and worries. But, I understood that he had to maintain his resolve, stay strong, and care for me. It was a terrible trade-off, but I knew he was making it with difficulty. We'd said everything there was to say to each other. He knew how I felt for him, and I knew how he felt for me. That he was here, constantly, seeing to me around the clock, confirmed what I already knew.

I shivered with a sense from the new and unknown I'd been feeling. A flash of understanding and serenity. I didn't understand it, but it was all consuming. I struggled to bring these thoughts to words, and when I did, they seemed so simplistic.

"There isn't anybody in the world I don't like," I said, almost as if I hadn't thought the thought myself. Almost as if someone else was saying it. But, I did say it.

Ray came around the bed and looked at me with the most quizzical stare. I wanted to explain myself, but I couldn't. The thought and the statement would have to stand on its own. There was no way I could explain all that I was feeling or seeing, no way that I understood it all myself. It was just there, and I was just trying to relate it.

It may seem that my telling of this is less emotionally charged than you'd expect; easier or more relaxed. It may be, and maybe because I've gotten used to the idea that I'm dying. You can't sustain the high level of anxiety and emotional pressure forever. I would have burst before now. I've just accepted my fate. Maybe I've even welcomed it, now that I'm beginning to get a sense of it, outside my life experience. After all, I knew almost a year ago that I would die, and it would be soon. So now its here, or nearly so. And, it doesn't seem as hard as I'd feared. There's so much that I'm learning.

Chapter Eleven

I grew up next to a large family named the Mulloleys. I told you about the daughters who'd sung at mom's birthday party. And, I told you about the brothers John and Gerard, and how they'd both died young. I was thinking a lot about those times and those people, in a sense living again my life.

Kit had been here several days, I'm not sure how many, and I knew she was leaving soon. But for now, she was near my bed, sitting in the chair Ray likes to sit in. I could sense that she was watching me closely. I knew I'd withdrawn from them, not by choice, but because I just couldn't manage like I would have liked. They talked, in low tones, and I couldn't really hear them. I just knew they both were there.

Like I said, my mind was on childhood times, and it seemed so real. It was intermixed with this new, unexplainable field of sensations and understanding that I told you about: liking everyone in the world, for instance. That knowing that we were all one somehow. A peaceful feeling. Now that dad had told me what I most needed to hear, and my sister had come and been with me around the clock for days, I was at peace.

What happened now I can't explain. It wasn't exactly my childhood memories, and it wasn't the now that Kit and Ray were in. In this new understanding that I was learning, John Mulloley came to me. He just walked up to me laying in this bed, and his face lit up with recognition and he put his hand out to me.

"John Mulloley came to find me," I whispered aloud, needing to tell them what I was seeing.

I could hear Kit draw a breath, and Ray move closer to me.

"Did you hear that?" Kit asked Ray, her voice quavering.

"Yes," Ray whispered simply.

*****

I know it was Friday. I think Ray told me. Patience came to see me, and I welcomed her, but couldn't answer her when she spoke to me.

Kit and Ray had been talking quietly in the kitchen before she came, and while I couldn't hear all their words, I heard Kit ask Ray if he'd considered calling a priest for me. She said she was worried that I hadn't been anointed.

Patience asked me if I wanted a priest; should she call for one. If I did, just squeeze her hand.

It seemed right that a priest would come, and say things for me and with me that I'd grown up believing. I squeezed her hand as best I could, and I know she felt it.

It was still Friday, I'm sure, when I heard Ray's mom talking to him, and then by my bed and talking to me. I couldn't answer her.

And then a priest was there too.

Ray bent down from behind the head of the bed, his mouth close to my ear, and quietly told me what I was to say to the priest, and when. I mouthed the words, but nothing came out. The familiar verses swam through me, and I mouthed the responses. The priest touched my forehead with scented oil on his fingers, and blessed me and my soul.

It did comfort me. I hadn't believed in the church for some years, but still the words comforted me, and the priest's promise that I was blessed seemed to blend with what I had been experiencing these past days.

I heard Ray's mom talking with him, Kit, and the priest in the living room. She was saying how grateful she was she'd come today, how reassuring and beautiful the priest's words were. I heard Kit tell Ray how much she and my family appreciated his calling the priest. And, I heard the priest tell Ray that he could call him anytime.

Then the nurse was there. She put a catheter in me, and I felt the easy release of the little fluid in my bladder. I hadn't had anything to drink all day, or food for days. Still, my stomach cramped from feeling over full, and the nurse rolled me over and pushed her fingers up in me, and pulled loose what had compacted in my bowels. I knew all these things weren't working, hadn't been working, but I hadn't thought about it. Only how dry my mouth seemed. Ray or Kit put ice to my lips, but my tongue wouldn't lick the moisture, so it ran down my cheek. I could feel all this, but I couldn't change it.

*****

I know a night had passed, and I knew my stomach still cramped some. My mouth was still dry, and I hadn't moved at all. Somewhere people were talking, but I was mostly in this new place I was learning about and didn't seem to really care what went on around me.

Another night passed, I think, but I didn't pay any attention. Kit had gone, that morning I think, and now I could only sense Ray in the room with me. I felt the pressure of his hand on mine, but my skin didn't feel his touch.

Daylight filtered through my eyelids, and I breathed once deeply, then I slipped away from Ray, and this world, and this life.

Epilogue

Madonna Anna (Rose) West, Donna, died on a sunny Sunday afternoon, October 20, 2002, at 4:30 p.m. She was at home in her favorite room, our den, in a hospital bed that Hospice had provided, replacing the sofa under the window, and in front of the fireplace. I knelt by her, holding her left hand in my left hand, gently stroking her forehead with my right, as she breathed her last three labored breaths, some two minutes apart. Her favorite artist, Enya, played on the CD with "Only Time" softly filling our home. That, and a bagpiper playing "Amazing Grace", were the songs that celebrated her life at her memorial service that following Friday.

I ached to tell her I loved her, and beg her not go. But I was afraid I would crumble when she needed me most. Instead, I held her, watched her, and felt the final gentle wash of her breath upon my face. Her final gift.

When the funeral home came to take her away, they asked if I wanted a sheet over her head. I said that I wanted the sun on her face as she left her home.

My life ended that day. I have existed since then only to write this book, and to paint the painting of her that would share her beauty and grace with generations to come. Both tasks have been completed. I pray she approves.